Yoga for Christians

A Christ-Centered Approach
to Physical and Spiritual Health

Susan Bordenkircher

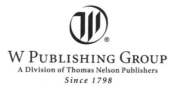

W PUBLISHING GROUP
A Division of Thomas Nelson Publishers
Since 1798

www.wpublishinggroup.com

Published by W Publishing Group, a division of Thomas Nelson, Inc., P.O. Box 141000, Nashville, TN 37214

W Publishing Group books may be purchased in bulk for educational, business, fund-raising, or sales promotional use. For information, please e-mail SpecialMarkets@ThomasNelson.com.

Cover Design: Becky Brawner
Cover Photo: Tucker Dorsey
Interior Photos: Jubilee Photography
Interior Design: Stacy Clark

Library of Congress Cataloging-in-Publication Data

Bordenkircher, Susan.
    Yoga for Christians : a Christ-centered approach to physical and spiritual health / Susan Bordenkircher.
      p. cm.
Includes bibliographical references.
    ISBN 0-8499-1270-9
    1. Yoga—Miscellanea. 2. Spiritual life. 3. Health—Religious aspects—Christianity. I. Title.
RA781.7.B67 2006
613.7'046—dc22

2005036492

Printed in the United States of America

06 07 08 09 10 RRD 9 8 7 6 5 4 3 2 1

To my husband, Greg, who always believes in me.

To my boys, Ty and Trent, who are incredible gifts from God.

And to my heavenly Father, who dreams far bigger dreams

for me than I ever dreamed for myself.

Contents

Part 1: Foundation

Part 2: Postures

Part 3: Stillness

Part 4: Application

Acknowledgments

I AM SO THANKFUL THAT GOD INVITED ME TO BE A PART OF THE MINISTRY OF CHRIST-centered yoga. Through this ministry, God has provided amazing opportunities to share Christ with people everywhere.

Thanks to everyone who trusted me enough to become a vehicle of support for this project, especially my devoted fan club of Greg, Ty, and Trent. Thanks for believing in me even before you fully understood what I was doing.

Thanks to my church family at Jubilee Shores United Methodist Church, particularly Pastor Bill Kierce, who allowed the seed of this ministry to germinate. I am grateful to be a part of such a God-led church body.

Thanks to Suzanne Winston and Pam Denham for taking a step of faith to establish Outstretched, Inc., and to Suzanne for remaining faithful through both famine and plenty. I look forward to all that God has in store for us.

Thanks to Greg Daniel and everyone at W Publishing Group for trusting me with the writing of this book. I appreciate the opportunity you have given me to share what I love to do and what I know God is blessing.

Thanks to Tucker Dorsey for the wonderful photography. Thanks for your and Susan's friendship and for letting God use you as part of this ministry.

Thank you, Jessica Bunch, for sharing yourself to demonstrate postures for the book.

Thank you to all my students who remain so faithful, class after class. Thank you for helping me grow both in my practice and my walk with God. Your effort and enthusiasm challenge me to greater heights.

Thanks to Trish McMillan, who "taught me everything I know" about leading classes and who inspired me to pursue a career in fitness.

Thanks to my support team of friends—Mimi, Elaine, my wonderful small group, and many others—who encouraged me every time I would begin to forget that "it's not about me."

Thanks to my family, whom I dearly love, for preparing me for this journey. Thank you, Mother, for showing me the value of a Christian home.

And finally, all thanks to my Savior, Jesus Christ, from whom I find my meaning. May You continue to challenge me to reprioritize and simplify until You are my one and only Center.

Introduction

God is using yoga. I believe with all my heart that God is creating a movement of Christ-centered yoga as a way to meet us where we are. God is using our desire to have strong, healthy bodies and presenting us with an opportunity to, at the same time, develop a deeper, more intimate relationship with Him.

My journey to yoga began with a seemingly random suggestion from my husband, Greg. He served on the board of the YMCA where I have worked as a fitness instructor for nearly ten years. As the practice of yoga was becoming more and more mainstream, the Y began to pursue starting such a program and was looking for those wishing to become certified.

I had never shown any interest in yoga, but for some reason Greg volunteered me to begin receiving the training necessary to offer the program. I had the same misconceptions, uncertainties, and fears that many other Christians probably struggle with when considering the practice of yoga. Sure, I understood the whole mind-body connection—I always have to use my hands when I talk. But bigger questions remained: *Will this Eastern practice compromise my beliefs? Am I actually worshiping something with my postures?*

I went to my first yoga workshop without a clue of what to expect. I'm sure that my attendance could have provided enough material for a *Saturday Night Live* skit. I didn't have the right mat, I didn't know the terminology, and I was dressed in workout shorts—which I soon found was a *big* mistake (Get in Downward-Facing-Dog pose, and you'll know what I mean!). But I quickly fell in love with the physical practice of yoga. It gave me a workout like nothing I had ever done before. It made me notice my breath and become aware of how my body was reacting in every posture. I could feel it working not only my muscles, joints, and respiratory system, but also affecting me psychologically and spiritually.

As a typically nervous, insecure, and therefore competitive person, I found that the regular practice of yoga began to change my perspective. I learned to get quiet and remain still. I began to develop a greater sense of contentment. I began to focus more intently.

But my greatest revelation was that God was using this new perspective for His good. Since I am a Christian, the quiet stillness that I was learning was creating a heightened attitude of worship and alert listening to deepen my relationship with my Savior. My contentment allowed me to experience God's joy in the midst of any circumstance, and my increased focus enabled me to get my mind off myself and onto something—Someone—so much bigger. Yes, my relationship with God was changing through my yoga practice.

I was so excited about this revelation that I wanted to share it with other Christians who struggle with health and spiritual growth. So I spoke with my pastor, Bill Kierce, about offering a class to our congregation. Our church, Jubilee Shores, is known in the area for offering creative paths toward worship, thanks to the heart for God that Bill was given. With only minor trepidation ("Can we call it something besides 'yoga'?"), Bill provided me an opportunity to offer Christ-centered yoga. I had no idea what I was doing; I simply knew that God wanted to use this practice to draw us nearer to Him.

Thankfully, at first, God blessed these classes with just a curious few, allowing me the time to sense what God wanted to do and grow in my understanding of the practice. But over a relatively short period of time, God sent many more students, and together we began to learn and grow.

Then in January 2002, my grandfather died. On the long trip back from Savannah, Georgia, to my home in Daphne, Alabama, I heard God express to my heart His long-term vision for the ministry of Christ-centered yoga. He made so clear His plan that it was literally like sitting in class and listening to a teacher. I even had to stop and take a few notes, because I figured if God entrusted me with His plan, I'd better not forget anything.

Two of the main truths that God expressed to me that day were:

1. This ministry is not about me; it is about finding a creative way to meet God.
2. God would touch people through this ministry, regardless of whether it experienced wide-based earthly acceptance.

With these truths in mind, the ministry of Christ-centered yoga took flight. I developed a video series with Suzanne Winston that has reached thousands. This ministry has opened the door for Christians to practice yoga without fear of compromising their beliefs. This book is another step toward helping Christians understand that God is using yoga as one of many creative approaches to get outside the chaos of this world and move into the rhythm of God's Spirit. In turn, I pray that it leads readers on a path to developing an intimate, real relationship with Him. Because no matter what the world tells us, *that* is what life is ultimately about: finding God, hearing His voice, and illuminating the world with the love of Jesus.

I feel so blessed that God has chosen me to be a part of this movement. It is unlikely that I would have had that opportunity if I hadn't been listening that January day, and I wouldn't have been listening if I hadn't spent the previous time learning how to get on God's frequency through an intentional practice of Christ-centered yoga.

Part 1

Foundation

chapter 1

Why "Christian Yoga"?

GOD CARES ABOUT HOW YOU CHOOSE TO TAKE CARE OF YOUR BODY. PAUL TELLS US in 1 Corinthians 6:19–20, "Don't you know that your body is the temple of the Holy Spirit, who lives in you and was given to you by God? You do not belong to yourself, for God bought you with a high price. So you must honor God with your body."

Those who choose not to adequately care for their bodies soon become enslaved by them. We become enslaved either by the desires of our bodies or by the pain and discomfort that result from lack of care. Paul is telling us that God's plan for our bodies offers freedom, since our bodies (and our lives) belong to God.

Your body is the instrument in which you carry God through your life. Therefore, taking care of your body is a responsibility entrusted to you by your Maker. Furthermore, it is a gift you can offer Him to express your love and honor. I encourage you to periodically take a personal inventory of what you are telling God by the way you care for your "personal temple." Do you respect the body He has given you? Do you value your body as an instrument of God?

You wouldn't purchase a musical instrument without some thought to its care and upkeep. My oldest son, Ty, recently received a guitar to fuel his aspirations of becoming a musician. He soon learned that the guitar falls quickly out of tune after use and that he must frequently tune the instrument for it to make the proper sound.

Your body is the same. If you fail to provide the proper tune-up, your body will also begin to work improperly. You will lose strength, flexibility, stamina, and balance. As your range of motion decreases, your ability and desire to do certain tasks will likely be affected. Your attitude may be negatively affected. As your weight increases (as is the case for most of us who don't exercise), your relationships may even suffer as you struggle with self-image and esteem.

Ultimately, as we'll discuss in a later chapter, the pain and discomfort you may feel in your skin can be the cause of division between you and God. How are you to share the love of Jesus, the peace of God, and the freedom you have through salvation if all you feel is uncomfortable and cranky? Do you exhibit freedom in Christ if you are bound by the limitations and inabilities of your out-of-tune body? If you represent Jesus to the world, what kind of message are you sending: one of brokenness or one of healing?

I think God will bless your efforts at exercise when you practice from a per-spective of healing. So if you enjoy walking, walk. If you enjoy step class, keep stepping. If you enjoy spinning, spin. All of these forms of exercise are effective at healing your body on the outside. And all of them, when practiced with Christ-centered intention, could provide spiritual benefits for the Christian.

An Undivided Life

However, I contend that there is no practice like yoga for integrating the mind and body in unity. Sure, the practice will work to heal the body on the out-side. Some of the proven benefits of a regular yoga practice include reduced stress and blood pressure, strengthened muscles, improved posture, reduced risk of injury through improved balance and coordination, healthier immune system and organ function, improved concentration, and increased flexibility and range of motion. Furthermore, medical studies have shown yoga can provide significant improvement for certain medical conditions such as anxi-ety, depression, asthma, diabetes, arthritis, carpal tunnel syndrome, and hypertension.

I could literally go on and on for pages about the positive physical benefits of a yoga practice. But what makes the practice unique is the correlation of the mind with the body in order to create health on the inside as well as the outside. To put it simply, the key is the breath. Your breath determines your movements and at the same time acts as the catalyst for a perspective change, a focus shift that results from the stillness and quiet. Add to that an intention for Christ-centered worship, and you have a recipe for wholeness.

For a Christian, yoga becomes meditation in motion, preparing your heart and body to work together as tools for worship. The Bible is clear in depicting the body as an integral part of worship. In Exodus 4:31, the leaders of Israel "bowed their heads and worshiped." In Revelation 11:16, the elders "fell on their faces and worshiped him." And of course, the Bible repeatedly instructs us to stand and lift up our hands to the Lord. He wants us to come before Him, ready to worship with all that we have and all that we are.

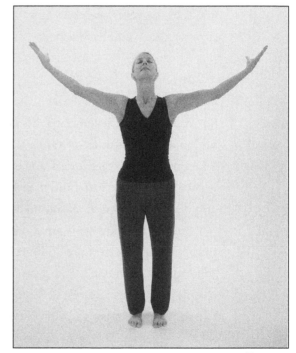

Figure 1.1

Matt Redman writes in his book *Facedown* that every posture in worship says something of both the worshiper and the one being glorified. "When it comes to expressing our worship, what we do on the outside is a key reflection of what's taking place on the inside. Out of the overflow of the heart we speak and sing, we dance and we bow. "[1]

When our Christ-centered yoga video series first came out, there was a lot of interest from local and national media because of the uncertainty still surrounding yoga in the Christian community. As I shared from the initial truths God gave me about this ministry, I was sure we would encounter some negativism. And God had prepared me to be content in the responses I received—both good and bad—because, remember . . . it wasn't about *me*.

But one comment that has continued to perplex me came from a Christian teacher who asked, "Why do we have to 'Christianize' everything?" First of all, I'm not sure "Christianize" is a word, but his point disturbed me. Doesn't God's Word tell us, "Whatever you do or say, let it be as a representative of the Lord Jesus, all the while giving thanks through him to God the Father" (Colossians 3:17)? You see, I believe this teacher is missing a key component of the Christian life. We are *not* told to compartmentalize our physical health, financial health, vocational health, and so on, with spiritual health needing attention only on Sundays or during our daily devotion. Instead, we are to live an integrated life for Christ. "Give yourselves completely to God since you have been given new life. And use your *whole body* as a tool to do what is right for the glory of God" (Romans 6:13; emphasis added).

Reclaiming for Christ

So to forego the healing benefits of yoga because it is sometimes practiced within a different belief system is like telling God that He is not big enough to take something from the dark and bring it into the light. Let's keep in mind that it was God who created the breathing process, oxygen, muscles, movement, and our body's natural relaxation response.

Some Christians who remain skeptical of yoga also question, as I did at first, whether the postures themselves are considered worship to something other than God. Didn't God create our bodies and entrust them to us as "the temple of the living God" (2 Corinthians 6:16)? Therefore, when you have a Christ-centered intent to your practice, how could holding that God-given vessel in any particular position be used for evil because of what another faith has named it? Simply because traditional practices use a series of postures as a salute to the sun, does that indicate that regardless of the intent of our hearts, that moving in those positions would change our worship from God-centered to sun-centered? Of course not.

Furthermore, suggesting that yoga cannot be separated from its Eastern history and therefore should not be practiced by Christians is like saying Christians can't enjoy the sunshine God provides because some religions actually worship the sun. Was the sun not given to us for life, health, and enjoyment? If God is big enough to make the sun, is He not big enough to discern those who enjoy it from those who worship it?

I love this argument in defense of Christians practicing yoga that was posted on the Christianity Today Web site by Agnieszka Tennant. She writes, "Worship is a conscious act of the mind. If it's busy overflowing with gratitude to Christ for the way he made my body, I simply don't have the mental space to give up to an idol. Second, can a non-existent idol snatch me away from Father God who has adopted me as His child? No chance."[2]

Called to Be Counterculturalists

It should be little surprise that God would use something like yoga to bring His children closer to Him. Throughout history, God has often proven to use people and things that the world would least expect. Jesus, our greatest example, was a radical counterculturalist. He turned the religious community on its ear, with much of His teaching in direct contradiction to what was expected. In addition, God chose to use Paul, once one of Christianity's greatest adversaries, to become His greatest missionary.

Consider the hymns sung today from most of our Christian hymnals. Many of those sacred hymns were adapted from bar songs that were popular at the time. John Wesley and others thought they could best reach people for Christ by meeting them where they were. So they took something familiar and turned it into something for Christ.

The same could be said of today's rock music. When rock and roll was first introduced, many thought it was evil and would lead to our children's downfall. And perhaps it has not always been the best influence on our young people, but no one could challenge the fact that God has also used rock music to influence the contemporary Christian music that has now reached many people for Christ.

The common thread in these creative ways that God reaches and uses us is *intent*. If our intent is to glorify God, to share His love, and to draw us ever closer to Him, He can use it. God is using yoga today.

Training for Silence

How do you draw closer to God through yoga? You allow the slow, intentional, meditative practice to train your heart and mind for silence. Just as a football player trains his legs for power or a baseball player trains his arm and shoulders for throwing the perfect pitch, yoga trains your heart and mind for stillness and silence.

When was the last time you were completely silent? No TV, no radio (even Christian radio), no conversation. No visual noise, such as thumbing through magazines or gazing at billboards. No emotional noise, such as thinking about your current problems or your to-do list.

Complete silence.

When you learn to become quiet and still, you are creating a heart that is teachable. David says in Psalm 4:4, "Search your hearts and be silent" (NIV). In silence, you can begin to see the attitude of your heart more clearly and recognize if it does or does not reflect God's glory. You can begin to see yourself and others through God's eyes, with an unconditional love that reflects the sacrificial love of Jesus for you.

A quiet heart allows you mental space to meditate on Scripture. It allows you a clear mind to raise up others in prayer. In addition, silence provides an atmosphere in which you can hear from God. He longs to give you direction, comfort, wisdom, and much more. How can you ever expect to hear a word from God if you never slow down enough or get quiet enough to hear His voice?

Joyce Rupp, in her wonderful book *The Cup of Our Life*, writes that "listening attentively is essential for spiritual growth. To do this, we need open minds and hearts, emptied of the clutter that blocks our way and crowds out what awaits entrance into our life. Listening is especially difficult to do because our external world is so full of noise. As we become accustomed to tuning out these external things, we develop a pattern of not listening internally as well."[3]

Train. Condition. Prepare. Learn to create an atmosphere that allows your heart and body to work together as tools for worship. It begins with silence, a silence that can be developed in a Christ-centered yoga practice.

What Is Yoga?

To fully understand yoga, you have to recognize that yoga began in India and is now part of Hinduism. However, it is *not* Hindu. It is a universal practice that is thousands of years old, predating Hinduism, and was not designed specific to any religion. It is considered a framework or guideline to direct people toward greater spiritual growth and physical health. Therefore, yogic principles and disciplines can be used in the context of any faith (or none at all). Easterners were simply the first to appreciate the practice's numerous benefits and apply it to their belief system.

Most Westerners have only recently begun to fully appreciate and understand how beneficial the practice can be. Many have chosen to practice yoga only from a physical perspective (called hatha yoga), eliminating any Eastern overtones or philosophy. Others have recognized the powerful spiritual element and integrated the practice into their own faith, thus creating the exponential growth of the Christ-centered yoga movement.

Early Yoga Teachings

Originally, the focus of yoga was much more spiritual than physical. Early teachers believed that to attain spiritual health, you must achieve all-around health. Practitioners were encouraged to train the physical body first, leading to better mental health, focus, and concentration, which ultimately led to a deepening of their faith.

These early yoga teachers developed the physical aspect of the practice by finding inspiration in nature (God's creation). They studied the behavior of animals and the patterns of nature to establish the original yoga postures, called asanas. They imitated the way some animals moved and found that the movements created strength, power, and agility. They studied the animals' breathing patterns and learned that those with slower heart rates would live longer. They noticed how plants and trees would grow strong and tall, with roots firmly grounding them. With this inspiration, early teachers developed a series of postures to create similar results in the human body.

After training the body, yoga's forefathers believed the next step in spiritual growth was to train the mind. They believed that an unfocused mind would not allow for growth or development. They believed we all have the ability to achieve clear, focused thinking but usually lack the training necessary to enjoy it. To achieve this level of concentration, they encouraged a focus on the postures, breath awareness, and an attitude of stillness and silence.

It was their contention that training yourself to concentrate allows you the ability to fully understand and retain information, to fully engage in conversation and relationships, and to be fully present in every moment. From this deeper level of concentration, yoga teachers believed that peace of mind was born. They believed that when our focus is fully engaged, our minds are clear of distraction, and our bodies are quiet and still, we achieve a contentment about life's worries and an understanding of our inner self, our soul. This contentment and understanding then ultimately lead us to the connection with our divine Maker.

Since yoga is a philosophy and not a religion, it makes no specific statement about a deity, nor does it require students to believe in things such as karma or reincarnation. Yoga is designed to equip students to find the inner meaning of their religion, understanding it on a deeper level. Yoga helps restore to people the foundation of their beliefs because it provides a means by which we develop the quiet, reflective, and receptive spirit that we need to be teachable. When practiced within the context of one's faith, yoga can restore to the student the intimate relationship with God that is at the center of our Christian faith.

A Paradox of Opposites

In fact, the word *yoga* is literally translated to mean "to yoke" or "to unite," representing the bringing together of one's mind and body. It also represents the union of opposites, such as energy and relaxation, or effort and surrender. These are all concepts that are integral to a yoga practice. Similarly, if we look closely at our faith, isn't our God a God of paradox? He sends His Son to be born in a lowly stable yet crowns Him King of kings. Jesus tells us that in order to be first, we must be last. We are to find joy in our deepest suffering. And the cross, a symbol of execution and death, becomes the Christian's depiction of life and freedom.

The mystery of God is one we will not understand until we reach heaven's gate, but on the journey to heaven that we call life, we can find wholeness and health. We can learn to become quiet in order to be more intimate with our Savior, and we can find the joy and peace for which our hearts have been searching. It is a gift offered only from God through Jesus Christ. Are you willing to slow down, to accept it, to relish it, and to let "your roots go down deep into the soil of God's marvelous love" (Ephesians 3:17)?

chapter 2

Getting Started

MY TWO SONS ARE AS DIFFERENT AS NIGHT AND DAY. RAISED IN THE SAME HOUSE, BY the same parents, their temperaments are nearly polar opposites. Ty, who is twelve, is a perfectionist, internally driven, and active; but he is disorganized and messy from all his activity. His motor runs full speed all day, and then he falls asleep at night literally before his head touches the pillow.

On the other hand, Trent, age ten, is very methodical and precise. He may not complete as much in a day, but you know he's made sure to do it correctly, keep it organized, and maybe clean it up a little nicer along the way. Both boys are exceptional athletes and enjoy sports of all kinds. Trent, however, suffers from a mild case of arthritis, and it affects how much "boy activity" he wants to do in a day. Although he stretches every day (a must-do for those with arthritis), he still never feels as good in his skin as Ty.

As their mother, I have the opportunity to accept and love Ty and Trent not only as blessings but also as unique personalities. It would be a grave error for me to attempt to mold one of my sons to become like the other. They think differently, they react differently, and they are made unique by God and for God.

As their personal yoga instructor (with more home instruction than they'd like), I've observed that their practice is also different. The way their bodies are made, the sports they've each chosen to play, and their general temperament on any given day all affect their yoga practice.

Such differences are also evident for each of us as God's unique, one-of-a-kind masterpieces. Age, physical condition, weight, flexibility, emotional state—

these are not deterrents to practicing yoga. They are simply factors that determine the way, the length, the intensity, and the focus of how you practice.

There is no perfect pose. There is no perfect practice. There is only you, God's fearfully and wonderfully made creation, attempting to feel better in your skin, to feel clearer in your mind, and to feel freer in your heart.

Am I Ready to Begin?

With proper preparation, yoga can be a safe, effective, and rewarding practice that is suitable for students of all ages and levels of ability. Remember that before beginning this or any other exercise program, it is best to consult a physician to ensure the practice meets all your physical needs. Here are some other general guidelines to get you started.

Time. Try to practice at least three times per week to see progressive development in your muscle strength, flexibility, balance, and focus. In doing so, attempt to perform your postures at about the same time each day. This will help ensure steady progress and will help you develop a regular routine. Choose the time of day that works best for you when you won't be distracted by other commitments. For many of you this may be a laughable suggestion, since commitments seem to follow us at all times of the day. But pick a time, give the kids some crayons and paper, and shut the door. There will never be a perfect time!

Some people find they are stiff first thing in the morning, but our minds are usually clearer and energy levels higher at this time of day. Remember, Jesus usually picked the morning as His time to get quiet with God. At the end of the day you may have less energy and more on your mind, but you will probably find the postures easier because your muscles and joints will be looser. Choosing to practice at the end of the day has proven effective in helping students unwind from their day and improve the quality of their sleep. No matter what time of day you choose, commit to be on your mat at least three times each week.

Space. The space in which you choose to practice should be quiet, comfortable, and preferably warm. Think of a place that you find serene and enjoyable, and either practice there or model your space after that environment. Your practice area should be flat with enough room for you to stretch out in every direction.

Clothing. Wear loose, comfortable clothing that does not restrict your movement in any way. Organic materials are best so that the clothing will breathe and your skin will stay cool. It is best to practice postures with bare feet so that you can use your toes to help in balance and to create better foot health. Be sure to remove any jewelry, glasses, and watches before you begin.

Supplies. (figure 2.1) The only supply you really need will be a sticky mat designed specifically for yoga. The purpose of the mat is to provide a surface that is both safe and comfortable. The "sticky" texture will keep sweaty hands and feet from slipping. These mats vary in quality, length, thickness, and color. Your personal preference and needs will determine which mat you choose; however, be certain that it has a tacky feel to the practice surface. Yoga mats can be purchased at many stores or online.

Brick-sized rectangular blocks are not essential but can prove very useful as you learn correct alignment in postures. They can usually be found in stores or online wherever yoga mats are sold. You want to choose blocks that are solid enough to support your weight but "spongy" enough to provide your hands a little give. Blocks are employed to act as supportive bolsters when, for example, your hand doesn't quite reach the floor or you need to relieve pressure on your hands and wrists.

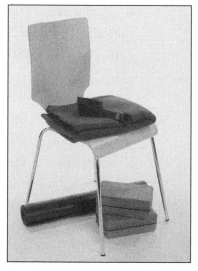

In the same regard, straps can also be helpful in ensuring proper alignment. You can purchase a yoga strap, or you could use a towel, sock, or necktie as a strap. Straps are best used when you are having difficulty reaching your feet or holding onto your leg. A medium-weight blanket can also be a useful tool for added comfort and support under knees and buttocks.

Figure 2.1

Level of Intensity. Most importantly, always practice

at your individual level and ability. On each practice day, take time to assess how you feel and at what level you want to practice. Always work within a level that provides challenge, but not pain. If you have particular areas of physical concern, be sure to know the appropriate modifications.

Pregnancy. Yoga is generally safe for normal pregnancies with the following exceptions: in the third trimester, students are encouraged to avoid twists, inversions, ab isolation poses, and postures that involve lying on the belly. Always check with your doctor to determine if the practice will be suitable for you.

Intention. Setting your intention for the class is essential if you are to use your yoga practice as a path toward creating a God-focus in your life. Using the quiet, meditative practice of yoga, you are able to view your life with more perspective and balance. You begin to see that the world's ways are not God's ways and to realize that His thoughts are definitely not those expressed by popular culture.

The key is getting your mind off yourself and onto something bigger. Paul reminds us in Philippians 4:8–9 to "fix your thoughts on what is true and honorable and right. Think about things that are pure and lovely and admirable. Think about things that are excellent and worthy of praise. Keep putting into practice all you learned from me and heard from me and saw me doing, and the God of peace will be with you." This means your yoga practice must be grounded in an intentionality that sets you firmly on a path toward God-focus.

While yoga can be practiced outside the realm of any spirituality or within the context of other faiths, your intent is what makes this practice integrate with Christian spiritual development. Tilden Edwards, in his book *Living in the Presence,* states, "What makes a particular practice Christian is not its source, but its intent. If our intent in assuming a particular bodily practice is to deepen our awareness in Christ, then it is Christian. If this is not our intent, then even the reading of the Scripture loses its authenticity."[1]

How do you make your yoga practice intentionally Christ centered? First, you simply change your focus. Consider this statement: *You are what you focus on.* If your focus is on yourself, even in the quest for spiritual enlightenment, then you are captive to your own limited capabilities. If instead, you keep your eyes turned toward God, you have the privilege of enjoying the unlimited power, unfailing love, and complete peace He offers. In Isaiah 26:3, we have the promise that God "will keep in perfect peace" those "whose thoughts are fixed on [Him]."

Remember that a Christ-centered yoga practice is about integrated growth, physically, emotionally, and spiritually. Therefore during your practice, you want to empty your mind of yourself, but not of all thought. This is one area in which a Christ-centered practice diverges somewhat from a traditional practice. In some traditional formats, yoga students are encouraged to use the practice to clear the mind completely of all thought; in doing so, they are supposedly brought into spiritual enlightenment or connection with their divine within.

But in a practice centered on developing your relationship with God through Jesus Christ as your Savior, your thoughts have more purpose and intent. You are training your mind to let go of self, to no longer expect to be the savior of your own problems, or to look to your accomplishments and acquisitions to bring happiness. Instead, you are attempting to use the loss of self as an opportunity to find God. You turn your problems over to Him. You give back your achievements to Him in gratitude. You stop looking to your husband, your children, and your friends to bring you fullness. You begin to recognize that the only path to lasting joy and peace comes from God through Jesus.

With less of yourself, you have more room for God. More time. More mental space. Fewer distractions. More awareness. Then, you can accept your appropriate size (small!) in light of the vast greatness of God. Changing your focus must be a deliberate practice. Your natural tendency will always be to revert back to a self-centered thought pattern, so you must devise a plan to take your thoughts captive for Christ. It is a relatively difficult task for most of us to accomplish (and relearn over and over), so don't become discouraged if your mind begins to wander.

Disciplines for setting and resetting your intention might include using a breath prayer (see chapter 3) or an affirmation of faith (see chapter 4) or simply allowing your practice to be preparation for meditation. In the discipline of Christ-centered yoga, you are preparing the body, the mind, and the heart to become receptive by working slowly and deliberately through your breath, your warm-up, and your postures. Then as you move into relaxation and meditation, you are able to use that receptivity to focus more clearly on the object of your affection and attention—your redeeming Savior.

In this method for establishing Christ-centered intention, your breath and body awareness become your focus as you lead up to the relaxation and meditation phase. As your spiritual awareness develops, ask yourself, "Am I connected? Am I paying attention to what God may be saying to me? Am I willing and obedient?"

Let the quiet nature of the practice calm your heart to listen. Let the awareness you create prepare your mind to pray intimately. Let these elements work together to establish a renewed focus so that you may literally "be still, and know that [He is] God" (Psalm 46:10 NIV). Remember, yoga is a very individualized practice. You are encouraged to work at your own pace and develop your own intention for each class. Set your intention for the class early, and let your postures and attitude reflect that purpose.

Finally, come to your practice each day with a sense of expectancy and anticipation. Anticipate that God has something special to share with you during your time on the mat. Expect that every time you are on the mat is a time for change. Enjoy the peace and quiet that accompanies your practice. Then acknowledge with gratitude to God the healing that takes place in you, from the inside out.

chapter 3

Connecting the Breath

GOD'S PRESENCE IS IN YOUR BREATH. GOD LITERALLY *BREATHED* LIFE INTO EACH OF US. Speaking to the people of Athens, Paul says, "He himself gives life and breath to everything" (Acts 17:25). He uses the breath as the singular vehicle for sustaining our human lives. "For the life of every living thing is in [God's] hand, and the breath of all humanity" (Job 12:10).

Without breath, you have no energy, no vitality, and eventually your earthly body will die. Conversely, with breath, you can experience renewed health, heightened awareness, a sense of calm, and freedom from the emotional roller coaster of life.

Your breath is also a reflection of your emotional state. Think back to your last anxious moment, such as coming close to hitting an oncoming car, finding that your toddler has disappeared in the middle of a busy department store, or speaking in front of a group and the "picture them in their underwear" advice really isn't working. Immediately, you react to this stress, your breath quickens and becomes shallow, your body warms, and you feel out of control.

Thankfully, God designed your breath not only to reflect your emotional and physical reactions but to change them. With deliberate intention, you can go from stressed to calm in the matter of a few deep breaths.

Most adults use only a fraction of their full breathing capacity, and the insufficient supply of oxygen is what allows stress and fatigue into the body. Learning proper breathing techniques will not only make for a successful yoga practice but will also enhance health, vitality, and emotional well-being off the mat.

Take what you would consider a normal breath right now. How much of your body "felt" the breath? For most people, a normal breath involves only the chest, with a gentle rise and fall. Now, close your mouth gently and take a deep breath through your nose. As you try this deeper breath, see if you can feel the breath flowing through the body in a way that reaches far more than the chest. Feel the breath move to the neck and face. Feel it flow downward toward the belly. Notice the energy that the breath creates, revitalizing your entire body. Notice also the release of tension that the deep breath allows.

Since your breath is what connects your mind to your body, that breath then becomes the single most important factor in maximizing your body's potential. If your breath is shallow and rapid, your muscles will not have the energy necessary to complete the practice, and you will remain tense and fatigued. However, if you are able to reset your breathing patterns to a steady, rhythmic cycle of inhalations and exhalations, you will begin to feel your resistance fall away, your muscles energized, and your joints open and receptive to greater range of motion. With every inhalation you are literally bringing in new life, and with each exhalation you are letting go of the old baggage that weighed you down. Eventually, you will learn to couple your movements with your breath until they are flowing in unison in a dance of movement and meditation.

Breathing in the Holy Spirit

Not only is your breath the foundation for your physical and emotional health, but it is also your gateway to actually feeling the Holy Spirit moving and working within you. As a Christian, God's presence is only as far away as your breath. In fact, in both the Old and New Testaments, the word translated "spirit" means "breath." The breath is absolutely essential to the body, just as the spirit is absolutely essential to the soul.

Your breath never leaves you. You may change your connection to your breath by paying closer attention to it, deepening it, or changing its pace. But all the same, your breath is always part of who you are. As a Christian, the Holy

Spirit is always with you as well. He fills you whether you are in church or the grocery store. He dwells with you when you are awake and asleep. The difference is your consciousness or attentiveness to that presence. Your breath can become your tangible, physical opportunity to wake up to God's presence, to notice how He is interacting daily in your life, to appreciate His majesty, and to accept His gift of wholeness.

Inhale deeply again, this time noticing the life that flows through you. That breath and every positive reaction it creates for your body is of God. His perfect plan is that our bodies work efficiently and properly, although that is not always the reality of our lives. After creating you as a masterpiece, God left behind for every believer a counselor and a guide. Jesus presented this gift after His crucifixion when He appeared to those who were in the Upper Room and said, "Peace be with you. As the Father has sent me, so I send you. Then he *breathed* on them and said to them, 'Receive the Holy Spirit'" (John 20:21–22; emphasis added).

As a Christian, each time you take a breath you are breathing in new life, the abundant life promised you by God, served out for you through Jesus Christ, and remaining in you with the Holy Spirit. Each breath is a gift and an opportunity for you to have a closer relationship with God. Each inhalation will provide the opportunity for you to feel that life, that abiding presence, while each exhalation allows you to release, surrender, and relinquish.

Every time you exhale, choose to turn over to God the things that weigh you down. Doing so doesn't mean your problems will miraculously disappear, although God certainly has the capability to eliminate all our problems. (We would just create new ones, anyway.) Instead, He gives you the mechanism by which to surrender your cares and let go of your baggage. With that release, the calm that you feel in the exhale should mirror the freedom that you feel in your heart.

Inhale the Holy Spirit. Exhale everything that is not of God. Inhale the power that comes from God. Exhale all that saps your strength. Inhale the freedom that comes only through Christ. Exhale and enjoy!

Proper Breathing Techniques

Proper yoga breathing is essential throughout the duration of your class. Therefore, it is useful to start each class by focusing on your breath alone, before moving into any postures. Doing so will ensure that your body is warming up properly and that you have set a breathing pace that you will attempt to maintain throughout the session. Focusing on your breath not only increases the intake of oxygen as you inhale and eliminates toxins such as carbon dioxide as you exhale, but it also massages and tones the internal organs as your diaphragm moves up and down with each breath. Focusing on your breathing also serves to calm your thoughts and improve your concentration.

The breath we will use for the purposes of our regular practice is the complete breath. Begin by sitting cross-legged on your mat. Hold your spine as erect as possible with your buttocks situated squarely on the floor. Close your mouth gently, without pursing your lips, and breathe only through your nose. Obviously, it is very helpful to have cleared the nasal passages first with a vigorous blowing to facilitate the nasal breath. Breathing only through the nose is an important part of the yogic breath, mainly because it allows the body to retain all of the heat it produces rather than letting that heat escape through the mouth. Keeping your body warm is necessary because it allows pliability of the muscles, which aids in the process of increased flexibility and reduced risk of injury.

Even the slightest attention to breath begins that calming, centering effect on your mind and body. After you are familiar with all the instructions regarding the complete breath, practice it with your eyes closed to further develop that meditative spirit.

From the seated position, allow your nasal breath to flow from inhale to exhale without interruption. Make it the deepest, longest breath you can take. The continuous flow of this breath will allow the body to warm and loosen. Take about five breaths with no regard to anything but moving the breath in and out. Then slowly begin to notice your posture. Extend up through your spine to lengthen from the base of your spine through the back of your neck.

Pull upward through the crown of the head as though you have a hook attached to it. Continue to lengthen each inhale.

On each exhale from this position, think of isolating and relaxing each of the muscles of the face. Often, we hold tension in our faces, especially when we attempt something unfamiliar or difficult. Commit to yourself that you will make every effort to relax the face throughout the practice. (It's better than Botox for reducing wrinkles!) Stay with the face until you feel it has relaxed fully.

On another inhale, open your chest, keeping your shoulders back and spine tall. On the following exhale, relax your shoulders down away from the ears without changing the openness of your chest. Place one hand on your abdomen, just below the navel. Breathe deeply enough to feel the hand rise and fall slowly with each deep breath. Continue this for five or more breaths.

Next, place your other hand on your ribcage and continue breathing slowly and deeply. Notice that as you inhale, your ribcage expands and your diaphragm moves down to massage your abdominal organs. Then as you exhale, your ribcage deflates and your diaphragm moves up to give your heart a gentle massage. Continue this for five or more breaths (figure 3.1).

Finally, move your hand from the ribcage to just beneath your collarbone. Breathe slowly and deeply

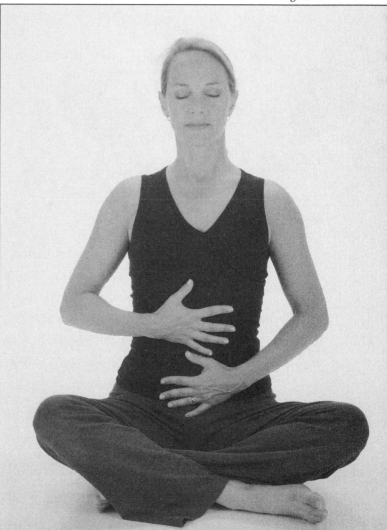

Figure 3.1

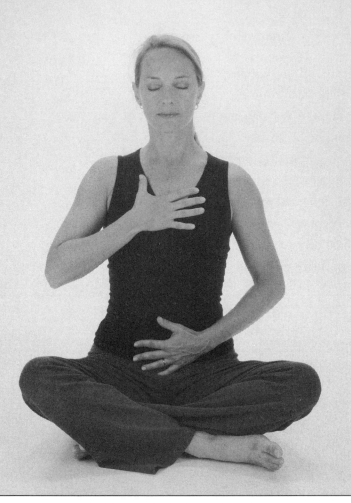

Figure 3.2

into the top of your chest, pushing the breath to the back of the throat on the exhale. Use your exhale to gently contract your abdominal muscles, drawing the navel back toward the spine and slightly up toward the armpits. Doing so makes it a little more difficult to take the deep breath but allows more power to come from your core, enables a more correct posture, and provides more protection for your lower back. Try to maintain these postural elements throughout the class, regardless of what other changes you may create through your poses. Take five or more deep breaths in this posture (figure 3.2).

Above all—keep breathing! The length and depth of your breath on both the inhale and exhale should be about equal to each other in this phase of the class. Remember, as a general rule of thumb, you lengthen and reach on the inhalations, and you fold, bend, twist, and close on the exhalations. As you sit, noticing your breath, begin to notice the air that swirls around you. Visualize God's love as the constant, purifying air that surrounds you waking or sleeping. Realize that that air and God's love are with you always.

Making Your Breath a Prayer

While your breath is the foundation of your physical practice of yoga, it is also the starting point for developing the quiet, receptive spirit that allows you a more intimate relationship and communication with God. Just as every breath is a gift from our Creator, so every breath should be a prayer back to Him.

Your breath can become a prayer simply by the quiet stillness in which you perform it, allowing God the time to speak to you in the silence. How often do we say that our prayer life is compromised because of inadequate time or focus? A quiet breathing pattern will provide both the time and the physical environment in which to get quiet with God. Part of that process will be an alert listening that you will develop as your practice progresses.

Richard Foster writes of this quiet stillness in his book *Meditative Prayer*: "In the center of our being we are hushed. The experience is more profound than mere silence or lack of words. There is stillness to be sure, but it is a listening stillness. We feel more alive, more active, than we ever do when our minds are askew with muchness and manyness. Something deep inside has been awakened and brought to attention. Our spirit is on tiptoe, alert and listening."[1] This is the process we are learning to cultivate by noticing the breath and allowing each inhale and each exhale to serve as a time of prayer.

While an active silence may cultivate a deeper prayer experience, so too will the use of faith words or a scripture coupled with the breath. Using faith words or scriptures should act as a centering tool to get your heart, mind, and body focused as one unit on the Lord. This type of breath prayer is usually not spoken aloud but spoken within the heart. The words or scriptures chosen should be short enough to correlate to each part of the breath. They should have particular meaning to you in your faith walk and to your personal circumstances at the time.

Considered a monastic approach to focusing, the key to using such a technique is in the repetition. One short scripture should be chosen per practice session. For further growth, choose only one per week, to be revisited upon every yoga session that week. Remember, use of Scripture is simply an avenue to get you focused for your encounter with God. The faith words or scriptures that you focus on shouldn't necessarily challenge you, but soothe and quiet your spirit.

Staying with this repetition is a commitment of yourself, a sacrifice of your mind's energy to focus on something other than yourself. This repetition, in effect, leaves you empty of self and open to the Spirit.

In *Prayer of Heart and Body,* Tom Ryan writes about this practice, detailing two of its purposes. The first, he writes, "is to lead you gently away from your own thoughts, your own ideas, your own desire, your own sin and to lead you into the presence of God by turning you around, away from yourself, toward God. The second purpose relates to the active nature of the mind; it must have something to occupy it. . . . So we give it one simple word or phrase to occupy it—a word which by virtue of the love and faith with which it is uttered, inclines our hearts toward God."[2]

As I've mentioned, choosing a scripture to focus on should be very personal. I have so many favorite scriptures that it is difficult to choose only one to mention. But I will share with you two of my favorites to help you understand this technique. I will list others within the context of each posture throughout the book, but for the context of this breathing technique, my favorite is Psalm 51:10: "[long inhale] Create in me a clean heart, O God. [long exhale] Renew a right spirit within me." As you breathe these words, you should feel the cleansing nature of this prayer for both your heart and your body. This scripture is about the longest you would want to attempt with the breath of prayer. The shorter the better, in order to burn the faith principle into your heart and to ensure it correlates properly with the rhythm of the breath.

Another of my favorites is Acts 2:28: "[inhale] You will give me wonderful joy [exhale] in your presence." Keep in mind in choosing your meaningful scripture that you are making this a prayer directly to God. You are speaking to Him in your breath. Therefore, choosing a scripture that is directed toward God rather than about Him will make the prayer flow more smoothly and naturally.

If there is a particular scripture that is meaningful to you but is not formatted easily into a breath prayer, make a simple translation to flow with the breath and to be directed toward God. For example, Colossians 3:15 reads, "And let the peace that comes from Christ rule in your hearts." Your breath of prayer may be, "[inhale] Let Your peace, Christ [exhale] rule in my heart." Simple and heartfelt. Let your mind repeat what your heart wants to say to your Savior.

Remember that a Christ-centered yoga practice is about integrated growth physically, emotionally, and spiritually. Therefore, we want to empty our minds of ourselves, but not of all thought. We are attempting to use the loss of self as an opportunity to find God. Make your breath the foundation of that process in developing a God-focus.

Tailoring Your Breath

Sometimes simply noticing and expanding your breath for several minutes can have a surprising positive influence on your energy level or emotional state. In addition, you can dramatically increase this effect by using breathing techniques tailored to have an effect on your specific moods and conditions. In an article entitled "Inhale, Exhale, Relax," Richard Rosen lists a few of the most common breathing techniques.[3]

Anxiety. You can positively affect your anxiety by focusing on your exhalations and deliberately and gradually lengthening them. For example, if your regular breath is six counts in and six counts out, draw the exhale out to seven for several cycles, then eight, and so on until you reach a length that works for you. Next, turn your attention to the subtle sound of your breath, particularly the soft "ha" at the end of each breath. Begin to pause briefly at the end of each exhale, resting peacefully in the stillness.

Let God calm you through His presence, using your breath as a prayer. Since the emphasis of your breath is on the exhale, a good breath prayer might be silence on the inhale and a long "You, O God, are my refuge" (Psalm 59:17).

Fatigue. To combat fatigue, return first to your regular breath. Then after the breath is smoothed out and slowed down, pause briefly after each exhalation before beginning the next inhalation. Rest peacefully in this stillness. After a few seconds, you will feel the rise of your next breath building like a wave. Don't give into the breath immediately, but instead let it gather and grow. After a few more seconds, allow the inhalation to come and repeat the process, gradually lengthening the inhales. Finally, try to shift your focus to the sound of your inhale. Try to make the sound, and your breath, as soft and even as possible.

This lengthened inhale is the perfect opportunity to use your breath as a prayer. In your heart and with your subtle breath, ask God to fill you with the energy, strength, and joy that only comes from Him. On each inhale, say, "Fill me"; rest in the exhale and enjoy the quiet stillness.

Depression. Working with depression can be a bit trickier than combating anxiety and fatigue. For that reason, be careful about how you apply the breathing techniques, since forcing the breath can make your condition worse. As with any breath work, start in a comfortable position and allow your regular breath to slow down and smooth out. Then count the length of your inhalation. When you release it, match its length to an exhalation. Continue balancing the breath for a minute or two, and then gradually lengthen both the inhale and the exhale. Start with a particular goal, maybe ten minutes, but always be prepared to shorten it if you feel depression lifting or to lengthen it if your mood suits.

To make your breath a prayer, simply determine what would be most helpful to your condition. Letting your mind rest completely and having God speak into the silence may be your best medicine. However, finding and reciting in your heart a scripture that has particular meaning in your situation may also be beneficial. One example would be using Psalm 37:5: "[inhale] I trust You [exhale], and You will help me (paraphrase)." Let the words come slowly and deliberately to match the breath.

There is no right answer in determining how long or how often you should practice these breathing remedies to make them effective. Like any other practice, the more you do it, the more proficient you become. The important thing is to just do it—whether for thirty minutes every other day or for sixty-second breaks at random moments in your day. Let these "Sabbath moments" be an opportunity to recharge your body, calm your spirit, and connect you to your one and only Savior. The results will be significant to your body and your heart.

Part 2

Postures

chapter 4

Getting Warm

BEFORE WE GET TO THE "MEAT" OF THE YOGA CLASS, FIRST WE MUST CONSIDER HOW we can prepare the body for the struggles and challenges of the postures we will practice. A series of warm-up flows (sequence of positions) is essential to ensuring you can attempt postures with greater comfort and less risk of injury. We began the process of heating the body with our breath and will continue to nurture that heat with some gentle movements and then progressively more challenging ones.

Think of your body as a furnace, which when ignited creates enough heat to fuel the entire body. The heat created in your body acts to make your muscles pliable, creates sweat that releases toxins and excess fluid, and releases pent-up tension. Reshaping and growth cannot occur without the internal fire first preparing the way.

Likewise, the process of burning away the internal debris of our lives is essential if you are to create the kind of environment that God can use to its fullest potential. Consider the trees in the forest as an analogy. Their ultimate purpose is to grow strong, providing oxygen to the earth and bearing fruit. However, they are unable to fulfill their ultimate purpose when the weeds, thorns, and underbrush of the forest begin to grow around them. If left untended, the underbrush will grow in size and importance, eventually stifling the growth of the tree and creating an environment in which the tree is unable to yield any fruit at all.

However, a skilled forester knows that if a controlled fire is set within that environment, then the underbrush that threatens the tree is eliminated. Enough space is created around the tree to allow its roots to grow and its limbs to spread. Ultimately, an environment is created from the fire that allows the tree to fulfill its purpose and provide the fruit it was designed to bear.

If your life is filled with weeds and thorns, you will not have enough spiritual space in your heart for God's work. The weeds and thorns of hurt and bitterness will grow in both size and importance. The debris of your life chokes you, stifling your growth and rendering you ineffective to fulfill God's purpose for your life.

When creating a space for God, you burn the weeds and clean out your heart to make it a place conducive to growth and health. Zechariah 13:9 offers this promise from God: "I will bring [them] through the fire and make them pure, just as gold and silver are refined and purified by fire. They will call on my name, and I will answer them. I will say, 'These are my people,' and they will say, 'The LORD is our God.'"

Wayne Cordeiro addresses creating space in your life in his book *Rising Above*. He calls it the "principle of margins," with margins being defined as the depiction of "the space between your load and your limit." He explains that if the load you are carrying is 80 pounds and your absolute limit is 100 pounds, then you have a 20 percent margin. If you are carrying 100 pounds when your limit is 100 pounds, then "you are marginless or at capacity."

Cordeiro says, "One reason you may live in such complexity is because you are living a marginless life. Crowdedness creeps in unnoticed and grows like aggressive ground cover till it takes over your life and demands allegiance. A marginless life leaves us no opportunity to develop relationships, no time to spend with God, and no chance to hear His quiet whisper."[1]

We create wider life margins by simplifying our lives, pruning back the ground cover that threatens our fruitfulness. We can simplify our daily schedules and our overwhelming responsibilities, but we can also prune away the thorns and weeds that congest our minds. We can cut away the tangled vines by turning over our hurts, our worries, and our personal agendas to the Master Scheduler.

How to Create Space

Again, your goal is to correlate the flow of your breath, the movements of your body, and the thoughts of your mind into a prayer of your heart. With each breath and each movement, you are trying to create both physical and spiritual space.

Since each inhale allows for expansion and lengthening, you will attempt to create space during that part of each breath. Think back to the breathing cues and posturing as an example. You are to use the inhalation to lengthen the spine and create an environment safe for movement. Therefore, you are creating space in your back. At the same time, notice how your chest expands and you feel a cleansing of your respiratory system. Allow that to translate into a cleansing of your heart and mind, as well, releasing the frustrations, expectations, and stress you are harboring.

On the other hand, the exhale is designed for movement into the space you created on the inhale. You lengthened on the inhale for the purpose of creating space and then moved into that new, clean space on the exhale. Think back again to the breathing posture. As you created length in your back, you were able to release your shoulders down from the high-tension position in which they are normally held. You moved into that space on the exhale. You didn't have to force or coerce the gentle movement. Instead, your body *relaxed* into it.

Being able to sink deeper into a pose is the result of learning to relax on the exhale into the clean space your inhale creates. If you hold your breath, you not only deprive the muscles of the energy they need to work, but you also deprive yourself of the growth you could experience as well as the relaxation that would result. In effect, you allow yourself to be stifled by the weeds and thorns.

As you learn this skill, a helpful tool may be to use a breath prayer that reinforces this concept in your mind and heart. For example, you could adapt Acts 2:26 and say, "My body rests in Your hope, Lord." On your inhale, simply listen to your breath as you breathe in life. Then on the exhale, express this prayer in your heart as you relax into the reassurance of that thought and into the physical change that is created.

This process of lengthening and energizing on each inhale and relaxing and deepening on each exhale should continue throughout your entire practice session. Let the breath and the subsequent movement be an ongoing reminder of your purpose and intent for the practice.

Affirm Your Faith

An outward expression of your God-focused yoga practice and perspective is to start each session with an affirmation of your faith. Used with repetition to begin each class, an affirmation of faith defines your intention and hones your focus. Of course, you may develop your own affirmation prayer to reflect any personal leadings from God. I will lead you through one here that has been adapted from Nancy Roth's Trinity Prayer in *An Invitation to Christian Yoga*.[2] Unlike the breath of prayer, this affirmation is spoken aloud and is coupled with movements of your body. It should be repeated at least three times. Try keeping your eyes closed gently to keep the movement meditative and personal.

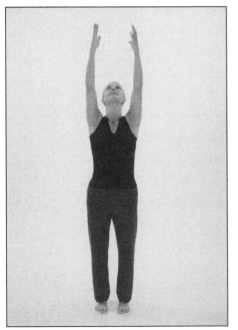

Begin in a comfortable position, either sitting, standing, or seated in a chair. As always, keep your spine and neck long and your breath deep. Inhale and raise your arms overhead until they are reaching toward the heavens. Leave your hands parallel to each other and palms turned in as if you are reaching for someone to embrace you from above. Look up toward your hands as you reach. Say aloud, "God, my Creator" (figure 4.1).

Next, lower your arms to your sides at shoulder level with your palms facing up. Reach your arms outward to both sides as if forming a cross. Keep your head in a neutral position with your gaze forward. Say aloud, "Jesus, my Redeemer" (figure 4.2).

Figure 4.1

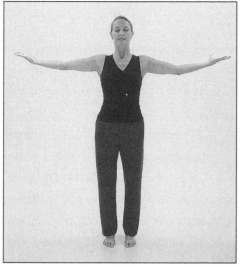

Figure 4.2

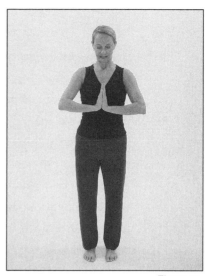

Figure 4.3

Begin to move your hands toward one another until the palms press together in prayer position at your heart. Turn your chin downward so that your head is bowed. Say aloud, "Holy Spirit, within me" (figure 4.3).

Finally, relax your hands downward toward your sides with the palms open and facing outward in receptivity. Say aloud, "I praise You" (figure 4.4).

Complete at least three repetitions of this prayer. Then remain seated or standing for several more breaths before continuing on to other postures. As you flow through your practice, if your mind begins to wander back to self and self tasks, come back to your affirmation of faith as many times as is necessary to keep your mind centered on God.

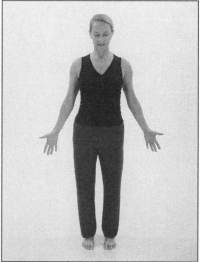

Figure 4.4

Limber Up

Always start the warm-up process with attention to your breath, noticing your posture from your comfortable seated position and the effect of the breath on your body and perspective. Again, remind yourself of your intention for this time on your mat.

As you begin some gentle limbering movements, pay special attention to any areas of your body that are tight or uncomfortable. Make sure you are attuned to how your body is feeling today. Let go of any expectations or goals. Instead, let your body work in incremental growth as determined by how you feel in each posture. There are never any "mandatory" postures. This is not synchronized swimming, and there is no gold medal involved. Your greatest "success" in this practice will come from going at a pace that suits you, avoiding or modifying postures that cause pain or restricted breathing. Limbering and warming positions are vital for you to practice before moving on to more difficult postures. They act to increase mobility in the skeletal system, invigorate your muscles and internal organs, and encourage mental relaxation and spiritual focus. Warming postures will also begin to build that heat we discussed by increasing the circulation of blood to the muscles. Furthermore, the gentle postures will loosen stiffness in the joints and begin to release tension in the spine. Generally, your entire warm-up cycle should take no less than fifteen minutes—more, if possible.

Start in your comfortable sitting position with attention to your breath (figure 3.1, pg. 21). Your comfortable seated position may involve sitting in a chair or sitting with your legs tucked behind you (figure 4.5). You might also choose to stand on some occasions to begin your practice in Mountain pose.

Once you have found your comfortable position, smooth out and lengthen your breath to the com-

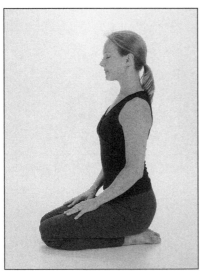
Figure 4.5

plete nasal breath. Stay with the breath until you feel your posture change and your body begin to warm. Make sure your spine and neck are long, your chest is open, your shoulders are relaxed, and your belly is firm. Breathe into your lower back.

Neck

1. As you are breathing, use your last exhale to slowly begin dropping your chin down toward your chest while keeping your back long and tall. With your facial muscles relaxed, let your chin drop a little farther on each exhale. Stay here for three to five breaths (figure 4.6).

2. On your next inhale, raise your chin back up, bringing your head to its neutral position.

3. From neutral, use your next exhale to turn your head to the right, with the chin pointing toward your right shoulder. Keep your face and shoulders relaxed and your eyes closed. Remain here for three to five breaths (figure 4.7).

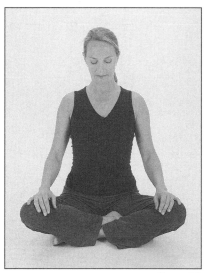

Figure 4.6

4. Use your next inhale to bring your chin back to the center and your head to neutral.

5. On the exhale, turn your head to face to the left, with your chin pointing toward your left shoulder. Remember to relax the face and shoulders as you breathe here for three to five breaths.

6. On your next inhale, bring the head back to neutral.

7. On the exhale, let it drop again toward the chest. Notice how the chin may have more movement downward now that the neck is starting to warm.

8. On the inhale, roll the head over to the right, with the right ear dropping toward the right shoulder. Make sure that the right shoulder doesn't draw up

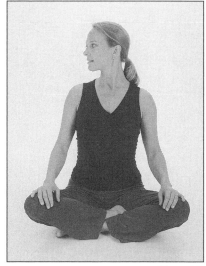

Figure 4.7

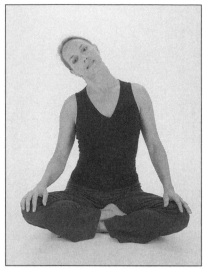

Figure 4.8

toward the ear. Instead, be deliberate in keeping the shoulder relaxed and down. Stay here for three to five breaths (figure 4.8).

9. On your next exhale, roll the head back down to the center. Use the next inhale to roll the head to the left, with the left ear dropping toward the left shoulder. Again, notice that the shoulders and face are relaxed. Stay here for three to five breaths.

10. Finish the neck cycle by gently rolling the head down on the exhale and back up to neutral on the inhale. Make sure your neck feels loose and warm before moving on to the next cycle.

Shoulders

1. With the chest open, the spine tall, and the face relaxed, begin to notice more intentionally the posture of your shoulders. On the inhale, draw your shoulders up as far as they will lift toward your ears (figure 4.9).

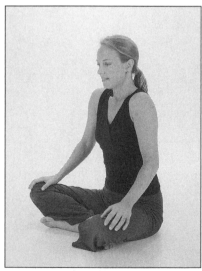

Figure 4.9

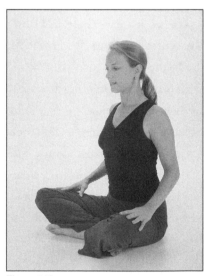

Figure 4.10

2. On the exhale, slowly drop the shoulders down to their fully relaxed position with the chest open. Do this three to five times, moving with the flow of your breath (figure 4.10).

3. Next, place your hands, palms down, on the top of your shoulders. On the inhale, draw your elbows forward toward one another, then upward toward the sky (figure 4.11).

4. On the exhale, finish the circular rotation by drawing your shoulders down and back until they return to their starting point. Make the rotations as exaggerated as possible as you circle them around. Make three rotations clockwise, then reverse direction for three more rotations.

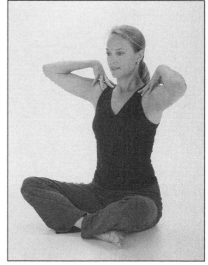

Figure 4.11

Feet

1. If you are not already seated with legs crossed in front, do so now to warm the feet. You could also choose to do this while seated in a chair if that is a more comfortable position for you. Reach down with the right hand and take hold of the left foot.

2. Rest the palm of your right hand on the underside of the foot. Use your left fingers to interlace a finger between each toe one at a time. Once they are interlaced, bend your fingers down to gently grab the top portion of the foot (figure 4.12).

3. On the exhale, gently squeeze your knuckles together to create energy and wake up the foot.

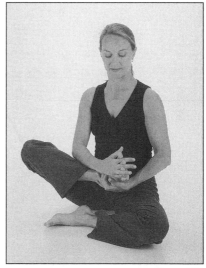

Figure 4.12

4. On the inhale, keep the fingers interlaced, but open the fingers and spread them wide, creating space between each toe. Do this three to five times until the foot feels more comfortable with this movement.

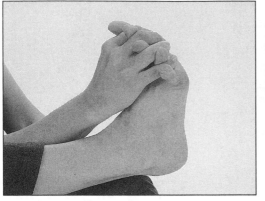

Figure 4.13

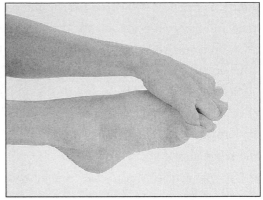

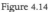

Figure 4.14

5. Still keeping the fingers interlaced, loosely hold the top of the foot and draw it back as if pointing the toes back toward the knee (flexing the foot) on the exhale (figure 4.13).

6. Use the inhale to draw the foot in the other direction, with the toes pointing away from the knee. Create this movement for the foot for three to five breaths (figure 4.14).

7. Release the foot by using your inhale to spread the fingers wide and slide them out from between the toes. Relax your foot down on the exhale. Repeat the same cycle for the other foot using the left hand. Stay with the foot until it feels both energized and stretched. You should be able to spread the toes without using your hands after you are finished.

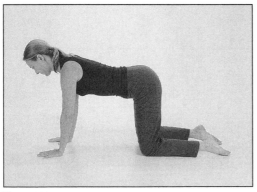

Figure 4.15

Hips and Back

1. Move slowly into Tabletop position, resting on all fours. Make sure that your hands are positioned directly under your shoulders and your knees directly under your hips. (figure 4.15) If your knees are sensitive, always have a towel handy to rest under the knees for additional cush-

ion. If you don't have a towel, try folding up the end of your mat to a double thickness.

2. Start by using your inhale to lengthen the spine and neck in Tabletop position. Relax to the top of your foot, and draw the front of your ankle toward the floor.

3. Use your exhale to soften your elbows, and let your hips drop to the right as far as they can go comfortably. Keep both hands on the floor, with the elbows bent and shoulders strong. Keep both knees on the floor as well. Stay with hips to the right for about three breaths (figure 4.16).

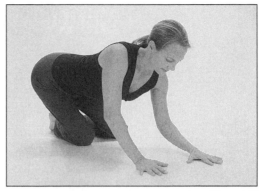

Figure 4.16

4. Use your inhale to return to Tabletop position. On the next exhale, drop your hips to the left side for about three breaths.

5. On the inhale, return to Tabletop. Use your exhale to arch your spine upward, rounding it toward the sky. Tuck in your tailbone and draw your navel toward your spine. At the same time, pull your chin under toward your chest with the head tucking between your arms. Think of it as bringing the pubic bone and forehead as close together as possible (figure 4.17).

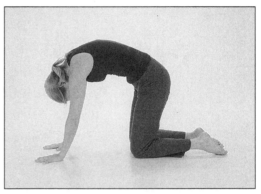

Figure 4.17

6. On the inhale, reverse the movement of your spine by pressing the back downward while the chin and tailbone lift. Look upward as the chin lifts and the chest opens. (figure 4.18) Repeat the cycle of opening

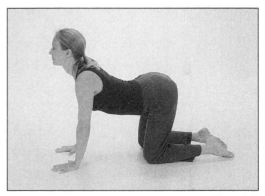

Figure 4.18

and closing the spine for three to five rotations. Always move deliberately, and follow the flow of your breath.

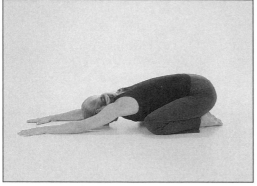

Figure 4.19

Now you are ready to rest back into Child's Pose (figure 4.26 as described on pg. 44) or to walk your feet forward to standing to complete the rest of the warm-up flow. For Child's Pose, simply lift your tailbone and sit back toward your heels from Tabletop. Listen to your knees to determine how far back toward the heels you can relax. If this is uncomfortable for your knees, roll up your towel or use your folded blanket, and place it behind your knees for support and comfort. Hinge from the hips as you fold the upper body down to rest on or near the thighs. Rest your forehead on the floor or on a folded blanket. Let the arms extend out overhead to encourage lengthening of the spine and create length in the side body. Keep your palms facing down, elbows soft.

Warm-Up Flows

Deciding which warm-up flow you will do on any given day should take into account the following variables:

1. How do I feel today physically?
2. How do I feel today emotionally?
3. What is my intention for today's practice?

As always, it is important to tailor your practice around these variables. You may choose not to do either of the warm-up flows and instead move right to selected postures. However, be certain in doing so that your body is warm and supple and you are not pushing it beyond where it is ready to go.

Both of the warm-up flows are about awakening your body and readying it for practice. The main difference between the two is the level of strength required. If you lack or are just beginning to develop core strength, I would suggest using the low-intensity flow. Continue with this sequence until you feel ready for more challenge, remembering that you may never choose to move on to high-intensity flows—and that's OK!

The flow of postures is a sequence that is synchronized with the breath to work together smoothly. This fluid movement tones and revitalizes the body, realigns the spine, encourages deep breathing, and increases blood flow to all vital organ systems. It is also a dynamic way to ensure your body is stretched, balanced, and invigorated for the rest of the practice. In addition to warming up, you may also choose to integrate movement from the warm-up flows throughout your session to serve as transitions from one pose (or one side) to the next. See chapter 10 for more information about linking the postures.

Low-Intensity Warm-Up Flow

Mountain—*improves posture, creates a body awareness, and is a foundation for many other poses* (figure 4.20)

1. Stand with your feet hip-width apart. Your feet will be slightly separated, but your ankles and knees will be lined up parallel.

2. Root your feet firmly into the floor, with your weight spread evenly between the heels and balls of the foot and the inside and outside of the foot.

3. Lift your toes to energize up and out of the arches. When you are balanced on your feet, rest your toes back on the floor and breathe deeply through your nose.

4. Lengthen from your arches upward through your spine, your neck, and the crown of your head.

5. Gently draw your navel in and up, tipping your tailbone down and under slightly.

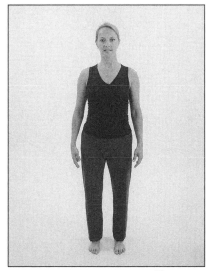

Figure 4.20

6. Open the chest, pulling the shoulders back and down. Your arms are active at your sides, with fingertips reaching toward the floor.

7. Keep your head centered and your neck neutral. Think about stacking one body part atop the other until you are aligned toe to head.

8. Fix your gaze forward, with the face relaxed. Continue breathing here until you are ready to move through the sequence of postures.

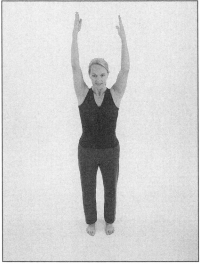

Figure 4.21

Mountain Peak—*awakens the body, lengthens the spine* (figure 4.21)

1. From standing in Mountain pose, inhale and gently stretch your arms away from your sides and overhead to Mountain Peak position. Continue reaching until your palms are pressed together above your head.

2. Straighten your arms until they are close to each of your ears.

3. On the first time through this sequence, keep your head in a neutral position as you reach. But on subsequent repetitions, begin to look toward the hands as you lift your arms, focusing on the thumbs. As you continue to warm, you may even begin to point the arms back with a slight backward bend as you lengthen upward.

4. Keep the spine long, the feet grounded, and the tailbone gently tucked under.

Standing Forward Fold—*restores elasticity to the spine and legs, improves circulation of blood to the brain and upper body, helps to relieve digestive and menstrual problems* (figure 4.22)

1. On your next exhale, hinge at the hips and drop your upper body forward in a fold toward the thighs. Try to keep your arms extending and your spine long as you fold.

2. Reach downward toward the floor, remembering that it doesn't matter whether you actually touch the floor or your toes.

3. Reach in that direction as you continue drawing the chest closer and closer toward the thighs. Forward Fold is a dramatic stretch for both the lower back and hamstrings. If you feel it only in the legs, modify the position by bending the knees slightly. This will give your back the opportunity to relax before you straighten out your legs again.

4. Draw the crown of the head toward the mat. Tuck your head under so that there are absolutely no wrinkles in the back of the neck.

5. Firm the belly and relax the face.

Halfway Lift—*lengthens the spine, tones the obliques, continues to stretch the legs and back* (figure 4.23)

1. On your next inhale, grab your toes (or modify by placing your hands on your shins) and lift your torso until your back is as flat as possible.

2. Try to lift your chest forward while at the same time drawing backward from the tailbone. Focus on drawing your shoulders back from the ears.

3. Keep your belly firm as you lift to protect your back. You may need to keep your knees soft to get a good lift from the chest.

4. Keep your head in alignment with your spine, again attempting to eliminate wrinkles from the back of the neck.

5. Keep your face relaxed with your gaze resting six to eight inches in front of your toes.

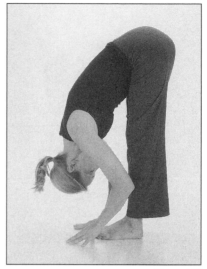

Figure 4.22

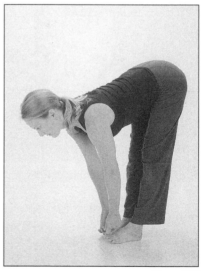

Figure 4.23

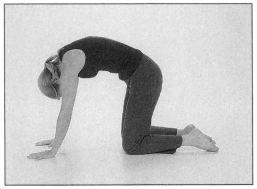

Figure 4.24

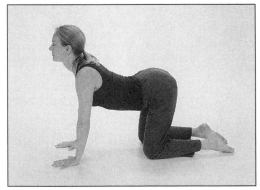

Figure 4.25

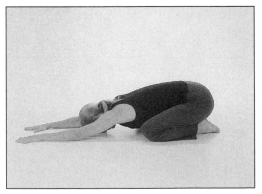

Figure 4.26

Roll Up through the Back—*lengthens the entire spine and neck, awakens the arms, encourages the circulation of blood to the head* (figure 4.24)

1. On the next exhale, carefully bend the knees and step back to all fours, or Tabletop. Hands rest under the shoulders and knees under the hips.

2. Roll your back up as we did earlier. Be sure to tuck both the chin and the tailbone under.

Roll Down through the Back—*limber the spine and neck, calm the mind* (figure 4.25)

1. On the next inhale, roll the back down toward the floor, lifting both the chin and the tailbone.

2. Expand the chest.

3. From here you have two choices: you may stay on the top of your feet and lean back into Child's Pose or, for more heat, strength, and stretch, consider tucking the toes and pushing the tailbone up into Downward-Facing Dog pose.

Child's Pose—*restores energy to the body; relaxes the neck and back; stretches the spine, hamstrings, and muscles around the knees* (figure 4.26)

1. From Tabletop, sink your buttocks back toward your heels. Listen to your knees to determine how far back toward the heels

you can relax. If this is uncomfortable for the knees, roll up your towel or use your folded blanket, and place it behind the knees for support and comfort.

2. Hinge from the hips as you fold your upper body down to rest on or near your thighs.

3. Rest your forehead on the floor or on a folded blanket.

4. Let the arms extend out overhead to encourage lengthening of the spine and create length in the side body. Keep the palms facing down, elbows soft.

5. Relax here, breathing deeply for about five breaths or longer.

Downward-Facing Dog—*encourages overall flexibility, strength, and toning; lengthens the spine; prepares you for other postures; encourages the flow of blood to the head; relaxes the face; relieves fatigue; improves concentration* (figure 4.27)

Figure 4.27

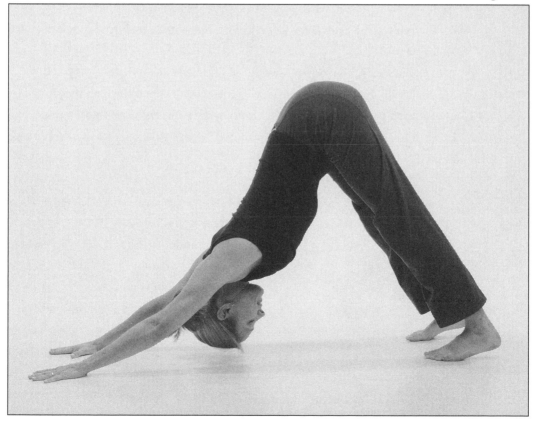

Downward-Facing Dog, or Down Dog, is important to the development of your practice because it engages your whole body. But move from Child's Pose to Down Dog only as you are ready and feel you have the strength to maintain the harder posture for at least four breaths.

1. In Down Dog, your hands should be about shoulder-width apart, with fingers spread and hands energized.

2. Use the fingers (and the middle finger in particular) to act as your upper body anchors onto the floor. Do not push down into the palms or wrists at all.

3. Straighten your elbows and keep them turned in toward your sides.

4. Use the tilt of your tailbone up to help pull your body's weight up and out of the hands. As the weight pulls out of the hands, draw it through the shoulders to the spine.

5. As you lift the tailbone, try to lengthen your spine toward the sacrum (lower spine), drawing the navel toward the spine for more upward lift.

6. Let your legs be as straight as is comfortable, with feet about hip-width apart, knees parallel.

7. Let your heels relax down toward the floor on each exhale.

8. You should form an inverted V, with the head dropped through the shoulders in a relaxed position. If you suffer from wrist pain, try using blocks under the hands to relieve pressure or trifold your mat under your hands if you don't have blocks.

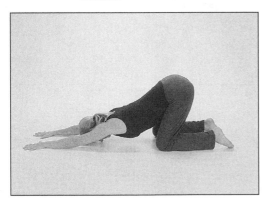

Figure 4.28

Half Dog—*same as Down Dog but requires less strength* (figure 4.28)

Another modification that falls somewhere between Down Dog and Child's Pose in intensity is Half Dog.

1. In this position, start again from all fours, but instead of sitting all the way back in Child's Pose, move your knees back about four to six inches.

2. From here, lean back so that your upper

body is in the Down Dog position, but you are resting on your knees with your tailbone high. Make sure you choose the option that is right for you and suits the needs of your body *today*. Always stay in the option you have chosen here for at least five breaths before moving further in your warm-up flow. Eventually this posture should feel both challenging and restful at the same time.

Tabletop Leg Lift—*transitions the body to lunge; opens and prepares the hip; creates length in the spine, leg, and side body* (figure 4.29)

1. From all fours again, move your left knee in slightly toward the right to rest at the center line of your hips.

2. On the inhale, raise the right leg up toward the ceiling, opening the hip slightly and drawing out through the ball of the foot. Take several breaths here the first time through, lifting a little more with each inhale.

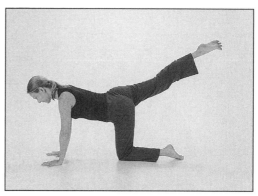

Figure 4.29

Lunge—*warms up the hip area, including the groin; lengthens the leg muscles; energizes the body* (figure 4.30)

1. On the next exhale, draw your right foot in toward the chest and attempt to place the foot at the front of the mat between your hands. This may take more than one movement. Do what you have to do, inching your toes forward, until you reach the front of your mat with the right knee lined up over the right heel in a 90-degree angle.

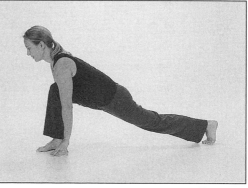

Figure 4.30

2. Complete the Lunge position by tucking the left toes under and extending the left leg back at a long angle away from you. Push gently through the left heel.

3. Let your hands rest on the floor on either side of your foot. Stay in Lunge for a couple of breaths while you awaken the hip, drawing your weight farther forward and downward into the hip with each exhale. Both hips should face downward toward the floor.

4. Remember to Lunge with the left leg the second time through the warm-up flow. Always alternate the legs evenly.

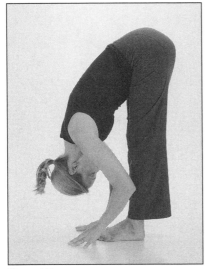

Figure 4.31

Complete this flow by using your next inhale to push off with the extended leg and bring both feet together at the front of your mat. Line up the big toes against each other and the outside of the foot parallel to the outside of the mat. Hinge at the hips and relax down into a comfortable Forward Fold (figure 4.31), with your spine long and neck relaxed. Use two or more breaths here to sink farther into the fold, allowing the exhale to draw your chest closer to the thighs.

To start the next cycle, bring your arms back as if they are wings behind you and lift from the chest to bring you back up to your Mountain Peak position. Remember that you will need to complete the flow more than once to adequately warm the body. I would encourage you to do no fewer than four cycles (two right lunges, two left lunges). However, completing more repetitions is beneficial since it allows the body to warm, the mind to unclutter, and the heart to still.

High-Intensity Warm-Up Flow

If you choose the high-intensity warm-up flow, you will notice body heat building much faster than in the low-intensity option. Therefore, it is important for you to set a good breathing pace and commit to move only with the flow of your breath. Remember to expand on the inhale and sink on the exhale.

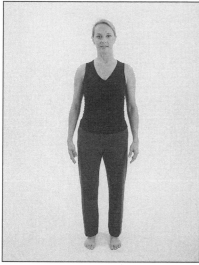

Figure 4.20

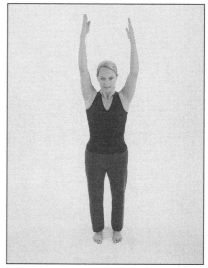

Figure 4.21

Mountain Pose (figure 4.20 on pg. 41)

Begin in Mountain pose, as described in the low-intensity flow. Take as much time as you need here as you center your thoughts, adjust your posture, and notice your breath.

Mountain Peak (figure 4.21 on pg. 42)

1. On the next inhale, lift the arms overhead to Mountain Peak.

2. As outlined in the description for figure 4.22, pay attention to keeping the spine long, the feet grounded, and the navel drawn up and in toward the spine.

3. On your first cycle, keep your neck in alignment with your spine and hands directly overhead. But as you warm up by flowing through subsequent repetitions, you can begin to draw your arms back, allowing the spine to gently bend and the head to tilt up slightly.

Standing Forward Fold (figure 4.22 on pg. 43)

1. On the next exhale, hinge at the hips and drop your chest toward your thighs in Standing Forward Fold. Adjust your posture using the description for figure 4.20, noticing in particular that you are relaxing into the fold rather than forcing.

2. Use each exhale to drop a little farther into the pose.

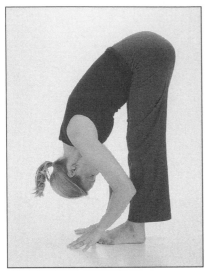

Figure 4.22

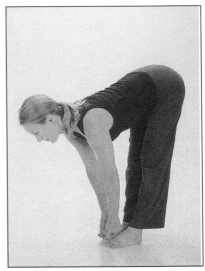

Figure 4.23

3. Keep your face relaxed and let your hands dangle toward the floor. On subsequent repetitions, you might choose to place your hands on your calves or your heels to draw the chest slightly closer to the legs. Never force the movement.

Halfway Lift (figure 4.23 on pg. 43)

1. On the next inhale, glance halfway up into Halfway Lift. Let the crown of your head and your chest draw forward as your tailbone draws back.

2. Use the opposing movement to flatten and lengthen the spine.

3. Rest your hands on your toes, or grab the toes and lift them off the floor as you perform this posture.

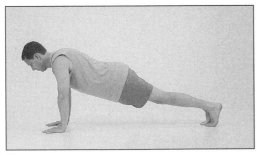

Figure 4.32

Plank—*strengthens and tones your abdominals, biceps, triceps, shoulders, and chest; harnesses your core strength* (figure 4.32)

1. On the next exhale, bend the knees and walk your feet back to push-up position. Create a strong plank with your body in a straight line, feet about hip-width apart.

2. Set your gaze below you between your hands. Make sure your hands are directly under your shoulders with fingers spread and the navel is actively drawing in toward the spine.

3. Let the ab control create a slight tuck of the hips so that the tailbone is pointed toward your heels.

4. Engage your quadricep muscles (the large muscles on the front of your thighs), and lift from these strong muscles so that your weight does not begin to sink. If you feel your strength waning, drop gently to the knees rather than let your shoulders take all the weight.

5. With the arms strong, keep the elbows tucked in at your sides.

6. Keep your face relaxed and your breath deep. The first time through you will want to spend a few breaths here to ensure your positioning is correct. On the subsequent repetitions you can flow through here rather quickly.

Low Plank—*develops core strength and encourages coordination of the entire body* (figure 4.33)

1. Using the same exhale (after the first, slower cycle), slowly and deliberately begin to bend the elbows, lowering your body toward the floor in Low Plank.

2. Lower your torso toward the floor until you are hovering a few inches off the floor. Your forehead, your chest, and your hips should all be equidistant to the floor as you lower.

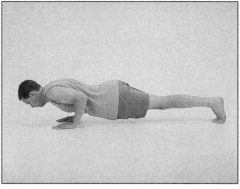

Figure 4.33

3. Keep the elbows tucked closely at the sides, so that you feel the arms brush the sides of the ribcage as you are moving downward. Notice that the elbows stay directly over the wrists.

4. Continue to activate and lift the quads as well as keep the navel drawn in toward the spine.

5. Attempt to lower until your elbows form 90-degree angles. If you feel like you are going to collapse, don't drop your entire body to the floor. Instead, gently lower your knees and keep the rest of your body in position. As a last resort, lower the entire body, but keep it in a straight line as you do.

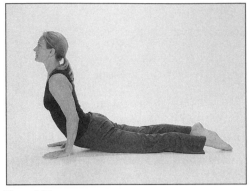

Figure 4.34

Cobra—*develops upper body strength and flexibility, relieves backache, opens the chest to encourage deep breathing* (figure 4.34)

1. On the next inhale, move into Cobra by pushing gently downward through the hands, then scooping the chest and belly forward and upward. This will cause you to roll over on your toes to the top of the foot.

2 Activate the top of your foot into the floor and lengthen through the legs, letting the thighs gently touch the floor without taking much of your weight.

3. Soften the elbows and relax the shoulders down away from the ears.

4. Gently squeeze the shoulder blades together to facilitate the chest expanding. Lift and open the chest, drawing the heart upward toward the sky.

5. Let the entire front of your body expand by creating length in your spine. Think about creating a graceful curve of your spine from your feet to the chin. To create more intensity, you may choose to move into Upward-Facing Dog rather than Cobra.

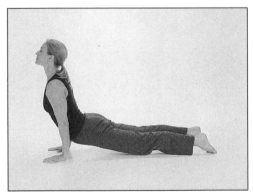

Figure 4.35

Upward-Facing Dog (figure 4.35)

1. Upward-Facing Dog, or Up Dog, is characterized by lifting the thighs off the floor so that the body is supported only by your hands and the tops of your feet.

2. Allow your arms to gently straighten out, without locking.

3. Be careful to keep your shoulders down, chest open, and face relaxed.

Downward-Facing Dog (figure 4.27 on pg. 45)

1. On the next exhale, tuck or roll the toes under and draw the tailbone up into Down Dog.

2. Use the power that comes from the thighs and the core to help you lift into the inverted V position.

3. Stay in Down Dog for at least five breaths before continuing with your warm-up flow.

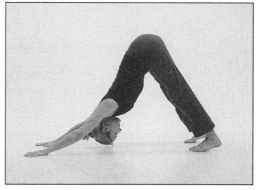

Figure 4.27

Down Dog Leg Lift (figure 4.36)

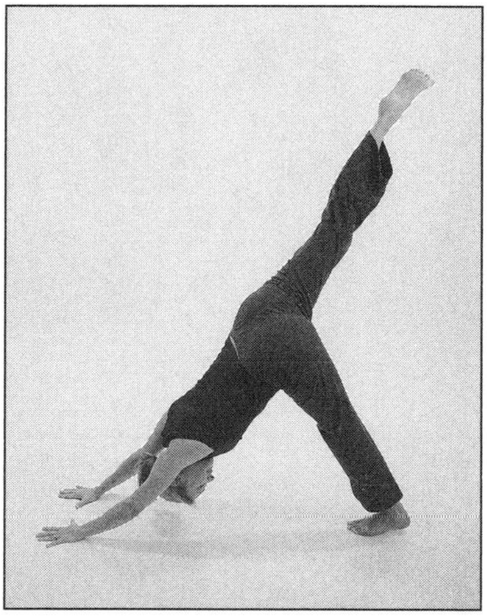

1. On your next inhale, move your left foot in toward your right foot until it reaches the center line between your hips.

2. Lift your right leg toward the sky, pulling outward from the ball of the foot.

3. Continue to keep the upper body and spine in the Down Dog position, with the head relaxed between the shoulders.

4. Think about creating upward energy from the right hip outward to the foot.

5. Keep the left heel dropping.

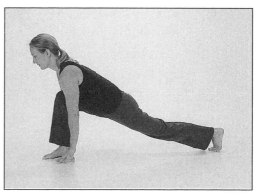

Figure 4.36

Lunge (figure 4.37)

1. On the next exhale, use the height you've created to draw your right foot in toward the chest and place it at the front of your mat between the hands.

2. Point the toes forward and draw down through the big toe.

3. Push back through the left heel, lengthening the left leg from hip to heel.

Figure 4.37

4. Keep your head in the same alignment as your spine. Stay here a few breaths as you use each exhale to draw a little deeper into the hip, being careful not to allow the right knee to push out past the right toes. Most of your movement should come from drawing the left leg longer.

5. Remember to alternate to the left side on your second cycle.

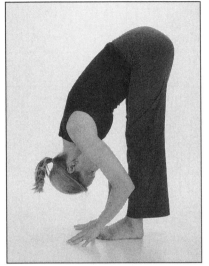

Figure 4.38

Complete the warm-up cycle by using your next inhale to draw the leg forward, lining up the toes at the front of your mat. Sink into a comfortable Forward Fold on your exhale. When you are ready to begin your next cycle, bring your arms back like wings behind you, lifting with a flat back to Mountain Peak. Do a minimum of four warm-up flows (two left lunges and two right lunges) before moving on.

Keep in mind that the more you do, the warmer your body will be and the more strength and flexibility you will experience as you move through the rest of the practice. Sometimes I like to challenge my classes to spend the entire session practicing warm-up flows, without ever moving to any other standing postures. The repetition of the cycles allows your body to loosen and heat. It provides an opportunity for your mind to be totally clear and focused. Consequently, your heart becomes open and receptive, on high alert to hear from God.

Ultimately, we are attempting to create space in our bodies, in our minds, and in our hearts. Use the heat of the practice to reshape the body, and use the heat of God's purifying fire to burn away the weeds and thorns that keep Him from constructing the inner sanctuary that we are designed to carry in our hearts.

Prayer for Transformation

"And so, dear brothers and sisters, I plead with you to give your bodies to God. Let them be a living and holy sacrifice—the kind he will accept. When you think of what he has done for you, is this too much to ask? Don't copy the behavior and customs of this world, but let God transform you into a new person by changing the way you think. Then you will know what God wants you to do, and you will know how good and pleasing and perfect his will really is" (Romans 12:1–2).

chapter 5

Finding Focus
(Balance Postures)

IN HER BOOK *HAVING A MARY HEART IN A MARTHA WORLD*, JOANNA WEAVER WRITES about receiving a birthday card that had a special impact on her. She writes that the picture on the front illustrated everything she was feeling that day. It showed a young woman with eight or nine hula-hoops swinging madly around her waist. Amazed at this feat, Weaver wondered how the young woman kept them all in motion. She thought about all of her own Hula-Hoops of responsibility . . . wife, mother, friend, writer, cook, cleaning lady, Little League mom, etc. . . . all of which made her feel as if there wasn't enough of her to go around. "I closed the card and looked once more at the girl on the front," she writes. "There were so many hoops, but she appeared calm. Her upper body seemed to be perfectly still, her arms outstretched slightly, as the hoops raced around her waist in synchronized chaos. Her face captured me. Looking straight into the camera, she smiled peacefully as though she didn't have a care in the world. Then it dawned on me—I saw her secret. 'She found her rhythm,' I whispered to myself. 'She established her center, then let everything move around that.'"[1]

All of our lives come complete with hula-hoops. We fill it with so many things that can distract us from that center, that place of balance. We become consumed with responsibilities, filling our days with busyness until we have no time left for study, worship, or prayer. God desperately wants to meet with us, but we're too busy for Him. So instead of centering on Christ and letting the rest of our lives fall into place around Him, we let our hula-hoops control us. This is how we ultimately find ourselves burned out, hurting, and disappointed.

It is the time you spend with God that provides a calm center in the frantic pace of your life. You cannot afford to be too busy for God, because it is only through that time with Him that true relationship is established. Through prayer, God can work, thus providing the peace, joy, power, and love that your heart is searching for. Paul understood this when he wrote to the Philippians, "Do not be anxious about anything, but in everything, by prayer and petition, with thanksgiving, present your requests to God. And the peace of God, which transcends all understanding, will guard your hearts and your minds in Christ Jesus" (Philippians 4:6–7 NIV).

When you begin to take the focus off yourself and develop a God-focus, then God can breathe life into your weary spirit. He can provide you the energy to keep those hoops spinning or possibly to relinquish the hoops that aren't necessary. By centering on God, your life begins to move at His rhythm, rather than the world's. As you move in the rhythm of God's Spirit, you can be changed. You can be used.

In his book *Too Busy Not to Pray*, Bill Hybels describes authentic Christianity not as doctrine or even humanitarian service, but as a walk—"a supernatural walk with a living, dynamic, communicating God. Thus the heart and soul of the Christian life is learning to hear God's voice and developing the courage to do what He tells us to do.

"Authentic Christians are persons who stand apart from others, even other Christians, as though listening to a different drummer. Their character seems deeper, their ideas fresher, their spirit softer, their concerns wider, their compassion more genuine, their convictions more concrete. They are joyful in spite of difficult circumstances and show wisdom beyond their years."[2]

In other words, their hula-hoops don't define them. Instead, their center, their focus, determines the rhythm of their hoops.

Balance Means Realignment

Balance postures in your yoga practice allow you to mimic the realignment of the heart's center with the centering of the mind and body. Without proper alignment, your body will not stay in balance. If your hips are not level, for example, you will tilt to one side. If your head is not resting directly atop your shoulders, you will lean forward. Attempting balance poses without the proper posture will leave you frustrated and unfulfilled. However, if you are able to first adjust your posture so that your body is in proper alignment, then your balance poses will provide growth and reward.

Your heart is the same. Until it is realigned with God's purpose for you, until you have the firm foundation of Christ, until you take your gaze off yourself and focus on Him, until you are moving at His rhythm, you will never have balance.

A great example of this concept comes from our class at the YMCA. There are mirrors that line the entire front wall that can be very helpful in checking one's posture in some standing poses. However, students quickly lose focus when practicing balance poses if they are watching themselves in the mirror. When the students' gaze is focused on their own reflection (or someone else's), then they are affected by every movement and sway that occurs. There is no firm foundation because they are relying on what they see in themselves or fellow students. Instead, setting your gaze on a fixed, stationary point (one that is firm and unchanging) will provide you the foundation you need for balance.

Balance poses are important to your complete practice, but remember that many people find balance postures particularly challenging. Don't become discouraged and give up on balancing. Instead, notice why you are struggling and find a way to work through those issues. Resting your fingertips gently against a wall or on the back of a chair can be helpful while you develop more balance.

I encourage students to integrate most of their balance postures toward the beginning of the class. Doing so improves your overall posture by making all the muscles work together, allows your thoughts to center, and gives you the opportunity to practice with muscles that are not yet fatigued.

Remember that you are born with a natural sense of balance (consider all the risky things you did as a child!). What compromises your balance are all the hoops of life that are swirling around you. Simply choose to focus and relax, letting go of all the tension your mind wants to create.

Recall the story recorded in the Gospel of Matthew of Jesus calling to Peter to walk out on the water to come to Him. What an awesome and frightening request, yet Peter was able to do it as long as his eyes remained focused on Jesus. Once Peter let his gaze fall, he sank like an anchor. Likewise, when we center our lives, our spirit's inner gaze, on Christ, He provides the firm foundation, the steady pathway, the constant rhythm for us to move forward with confidence.

Balance Postures

The two most important elements of balance postures are starting with a deep, flowing breath and finding a fixed point on which to focus your gaze. Use your complete breath to filter out distractions and to create a body awareness. Then pick a point that is stationary on which to fix your gaze. Pay attention to that point with concentrated focus throughout your attempt at balance. Make sure your focal point is at a height and length away from your body that keeps your neck in the proper alignment.

If you are attempting to create a God-focus in your yoga practice, I would encourage you to place some symbol of your faith (such as a cross or a Bible) at the precise point on which you plan to focus. A symbol can be helpful, but is certainly not necessary as you attempt to center your mind and heart. If you have chosen a sacred word or scripture, continue to repeat it in your heart as you move through this series of poses.

You may choose to do several balance poses in each class, or you may find one or two is all you want to attempt for now. Either way, be certain that you do the pose on both the left side and the right side to create proper alignment and equilibrium.

Standing Leg Raise—*creates body alignment and awareness, tones the base leg, stretches the raised leg, works the rhomboid muscle between the shoulder blades, creates focus* (figure 5.1)

1. Start in Mountain pose, with your hands at your sides. Fix your gaze forward, keeping your breath deep.

2. On your inhale, bring your left hand to your hip.

3. On the exhale, roll the shoulders down the back, while keeping the chest open.

4. With slow, deliberate movement, use your next inhale to draw your right knee in and up toward the chest, using the right hand to guide and stabilize the knee in place. Remember to keep your spine long and the standing leg straight as you balance on it.

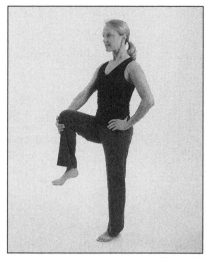

Figure 5.1

5. Keep the belly firm.

6. Keep your face and neck relaxed. If you find this challenging, stay in this position, stabilizing as much as possible, for five breaths, before slowly lowering the leg and arm on an exhale. Use your next inhale to begin the posture on the other side.

High-intensity option (figure 5.2)

1. If you feel you are ready for a further challenge in this pose, after holding the knee for a breath or two, use your strap or the first two fingers of your right hand to grasp your right big toe.

2. Lengthen your spine on the inhale as you lengthen that leg at a right angle to the body.

3. Extend the leg, unhinging from the knee as much as you can while still maintaining a straight spine. A rounded back indicates you've gone beyond your present capabilities.

4. Keep the belly firm and the base leg straight.

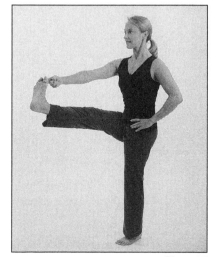

Figure 5.2

5. Keep your hips level and squared to the front of the room.

6. Relax your shoulders again on an exhale.

7. Hold for five breaths before releasing and moving to the other leg.

Low-intensity option

1. If the leg raise is difficult for you, try keeping your base leg slightly bent.

2. You may choose to use the wall for support.

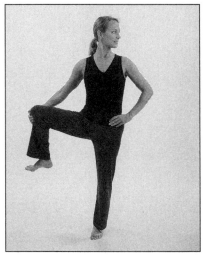

Figure 5.3

Standing Side Leg Raise—*improves balance, concentration, and posture; tones base leg; opens chest and hip* (figure 5.3)

1. From Mountain pose, shift your weight onto the left leg.

2. Bend the right knee and lift it toward the chest, stopping when the knee is at hip level. Place both hands on your hips.

3. Firm the belly, relax your shoulders, and fix your gaze forward.

4. Trying to keep your hips level and squared to the front, rest your right hand on the right knee and begin to draw the knee outward to the side. Try to create an open hip joint without changing the direction of the hip itself.

5. If you can, try to change your gaze to look over the opposite shoulder.

6. Keep your spine and neck long and facial muscles relaxed.

7. Stay here at least five breaths before releasing the leg and moving to the other side.

High-intensity option (figure 5.4)

1. Instead of reaching for the hand on the knee, see if you can connect the hand to the toe.

2. Lengthen the leg out in front first while holding the toe.

3. Slowly begin to open the leg to the side.

4. Let your gaze turn to look over the opposite shoulder.

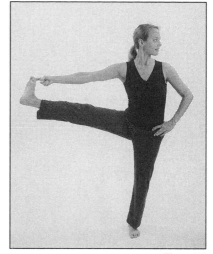

Figure 5.4

Tree—*develops concentration and focus, encourages an erect spine, tones the chest, tones the legs, loosens the hips, strengthens the ankles* (figure 5.5)

1. Begin from Mountain pose. Fix your gaze forward and keep your breath flowing deeply. Notice how your feet are grounded into the floor with equal weight.

2. On the inhale, deliberately and slowly pick up the right foot and place the bottom of the foot on the inner leg between the ankle and the knee. (Never, never, never place any weight directly on the joint.) Make sure as you adjust the height of the foot that it rests below the knee or, if you're able, move it above the knee to the inside of the thigh.

3. Press firmly down through the base leg, keeping the leg and your spine very tall.

4. Keep your hips forward and level as you draw the right knee farther open.

5. Bring your hands up to prayer position at your heart to engage the upper body and keep the chest open.

6. Your belly should remain firm and your gaze fixed ahead.

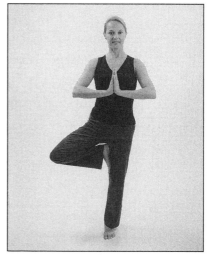

Figure 5.5

7. Keep your face and neck relaxed.

8. Remain here for five breaths before moving to the other leg.

High-intensity options

There are a couple of alternatives for you if you want further challenge in this pose.

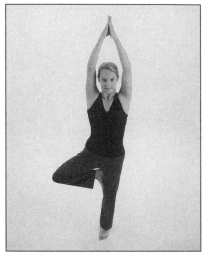

Figure 5.6

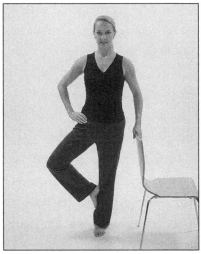

Figure 5.7

1. On an inhale, press your hands upward, lengthening the arms above the head. Press the palms together, with the elbows drawing close to the ears and the shoulders relaxed down the back (figure 5.6).

2. In addition, you can achieve further challenge by attempting this pose with your eyes shut gently. Be very careful if you choose to attempt this option, as your gaze is a powerful tool in your balance, and without it your balance will be severely challenged.

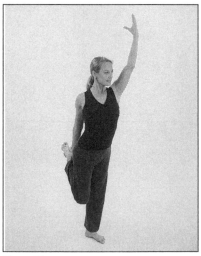

Figure 5.8

Low-intensity options (figure 5.7)

1. Keep raised leg low with toes close to the floor.

2. You may choose to use the wall or a chair to help in balance.

Dancer—*improves posture, increases focus, opens the shoulder, lengthens the quadricep, creates flexibility and strength in the back* (figure 5.8)

1. From Mountain pose, fix your gaze forward and breathe deeply.

2. With the spine long and the feet grounded, use your inhale to draw the left hand overhead. Bring the left arm close to the ear, lengthening the entire left side of the body. Turn the palm to face in.

3. On the exhale, bend the right knee and bring the right foot up behind you.

4. Use your right hand to grab the inside of the foot. Draw your knees in toward one another.

5. Keep the belly firm and the face relaxed.

6. Notice that the hips are level and facing forward.

7. Stay here and breathe until you feel the body stabilize.

8. Then begin to draw the heel of the right foot closer and closer to the behind until you feel the front of the leg stretch.

9. Remain here for five breaths before doing this pose with the left leg.

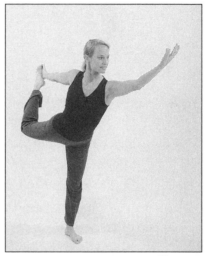

Figure 5.9

High-intensity option (figure 5.9)

1. For a more dramatic stretch and balance challenge, lift your chest and stretch forward, reaching the arm forward with the palm up.

2. At the same time, press the front of the right foot into the right hand and reach the leg back, drawing upward from the knee.

3. Let the hip lift slightly as you lift the leg.

4. Stay here for five breaths before transitioning down on the exhale and to the other leg on the next inhale.

Low-intensity option (figure 5.10)

1. Use the wall or the back of a chair for balance.

2. If you are unable to reach for the inside of the foot, grab the outside as a beginning point.

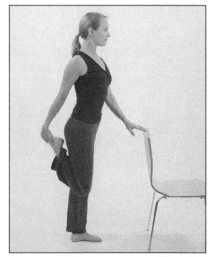

Figure 5.10

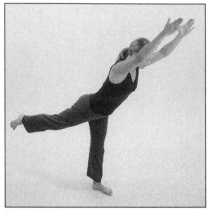

Figure 5.11

Warrior III—*strengthens core muscles, tones the base leg, creates a long spine, improves focus and posture* (figure 5.11)

1. From Mountain pose, notice that your breathing is deep, your feet are grounded, and your weight is evenly distributed.

2. On the inhale, raise both arms overhead with the inner arm close to each ear. As you do this, lengthen the spine and the neck without pulling out of the shoulder sockets. Let the fingertips pull the energy up and out of the spine.

3. Draw down into the left foot as you slowly and deliberately lift the right leg back. Keep the leg straight and lifting back as you keep the arms long and reaching forward at the same angle as the leg. Begin by creating a long diagonal from fingertips to toes.

4. Draw your navel in toward the spine.

5. Keep your face relaxed and your gaze in an angle that doesn't compromise your neck.

6. Create as much length as you can from head to toe and hold for five deep breaths before inhaling the chest back up to standing.

7. Transition to the other leg for five more breaths.

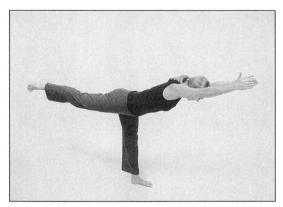

Figure 5.12

High-intensity option (figure 5.12)

1. Once you reach the diagonal, use the strength of your core to bring your entire body parallel to the floor, with your arms and crown of the head reaching forward and your hips, leg, and ball of the foot reaching back.

2. Your gaze point is now directly downward to keep your neck in proper alignment.

Low-intensity option
As your leg reaches back, keep your hands resting gently on the back of a chair.

Tiptoe Chair—*improves core strength and balance; stabilizes the knees and ankles; strengthens the feet, calves, and quadriceps* (figure 5.13)

1. Start in Mountain pose with your feet together and toes spread.

2. On your inhale, rise onto the balls of your feet and raise your arms out in front of you at chest level, palms down.

3. Keep the heels lifted as you exhale and begin to squat, bending the knees deeply. See if you can lower your thighs to be parallel to the floor without resting your buttocks on your heels.

4. Keep your belly firm and tailbone pointed downward.

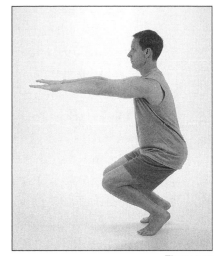

Figure 5.13

5. Be sure to keep your face and neck relaxed and your breath flowing deeply.

6. Hold this position for five breaths.

7. Use your next inhale to rise, standing on tiptoe.

8. Use the final exhale to release your heels to the floor and your arms to your sides.

Low-intensity option

1. Remember to bend the knees only as far as you feel comfortable.

2. If you have trouble balancing, try placing your fingertips lightly on a chair situated in front of you.

Tiptoe Straddle—*creates greater balance and core strength, tones the legs and feet, opens the hips, improves posture* (figure 5.14)

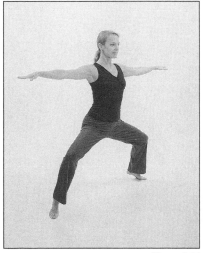

Figure 5.14

1. From standing, separate your feet three to four feet apart. From this wide stance, turn your toes out slightly to face the corners of the room.

2. Rest your hands at your sides while you get your posture ready to balance. Make sure that your back is long and lifting on your inhale.

3. Use the exhale to firm the belly, being very deliberate about creating a posterior tuck and letting the tailbone point down.

4. On the next inhale, keep your chest strong and raise the arms to your sides, extending outward through both hands, palms down. At the same time, lift to the balls of your feet. Try to keep your heels lifted as you maintain a tall spine.

5. On the next exhale, bend your knees into a squat until your knees are directly over your heels. Do not let the knees move out past the toes. If you can go deeper, adjust your feet into a wider stance to ensure proper positioning.

6. Stay in this low squat, resting on the balls of the feet, for five breaths. Be certain that you are protecting your back by keeping your belly firm, with the navel drawing back toward the spine.

7. On an inhale, come out by straightening the legs while the heels remain lifted.

8. Use the exhale to lower the heels back to the floor.

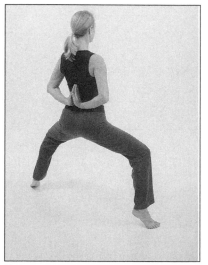

Figure 5.15

High-intensity option (figure 5.15)
Maintain the deep tiptoe squat while you position your hands behind you in reverse prayer. While it requires more balance to achieve this modification, it will give you added support for maintaining the strong chest and back.

Low-intensity option (figure 5.16)
Rest your fingertips lightly on the back of a chair to aid in balance. You may also choose not to lower into a deep squat but instead to keep your knees only slightly bent.

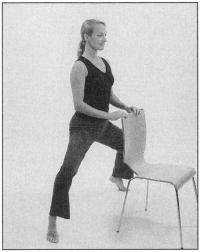

Figure 5.16

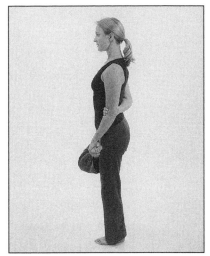

Figure 5.17

Bound Leg Cross—*improves balance and concentration, opens chest, opens hips, strengthens legs and ankles* (figure 5.17)

1. Stand in Mountain pose, with your arms resting at your sides.

2. Shift your weight to the left leg and soften the knee on the exhale.

3. With balance and control, cross the right leg onto the left, just above the knee.

4. Grab the right foot with the left hand, and on an inhale, stand as straight as you're able to while still holding the foot.

5. Draw the foot up toward the hip, with the knee pointing down toward the floor.

6. If you can balance here, use your right hand behind the back to reach around and grasp the left elbow. As you hold the left elbow, let the chest draw open.

7. Keep your belly firm, your face relaxed, and your gaze steady and forward.

8. Keep your hips level and squared to the front.

9. Try to hold here for five breaths before releasing your leg and arm on an exhale and moving to the other side.

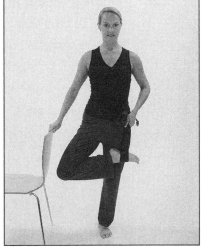

Figure 5.18

Low-intensity option (figure 5.18)

1. Use the free hand on the wall or on a chair if you have trouble balancing.

2. If you have difficulty getting your hand to connect with the foot, use a towel or strap wrapped around the top of the foot.

Practice Balance

Remember, the best way to improve balance is to *practice*. Consider standing on one foot while you cook, watch TV, or help the kids with homework. It will help strengthen the muscles needed for most balance poses and work to create better cooperation among your muscles.

Developing the focus necessary to improve balance also comes with practice. In addition to working on body realignment, set aside time to realign your heart and mind as well. Give yourself permission to simply sit and practice breathing and focusing. Use your sacred symbol to focus your gaze. Use your sacred word or scripture to repeat in focused prayer or sit quietly and let your mind become friendly with the silence. Just keep in mind that you cannot focus until your mind is free of distraction and your body is quiet.

What level of focus does God require? Romans 6:13 says, "Give yourself completely to God since you have been given new life." God's idea of a healthy lifestyle is not one that is compartmentalized by your vocation, your family, or your church. He wants the whole person . . . mouths that speak the truth of Him, hearts that pray to Him in earnest, minds that are fixed on Him, and bodies that worship Him. To do so means to intentionally arrange our lives around the goal of spiritual transformation. We do that with a focus from our minds, hearts, and bodies. "Fix your attention on God. You'll be changed from the inside out" (Romans 12:2 MSG).

Prayer for Focus

"To you, O LORD, I lift up my soul. I trust in you, my God! . . . Show me the path where I should walk, O LORD; point out the right road for me to follow. Lead me by your truth and teach me. . . . All day long I put my hope in you" (Psalm 25:1–2, 4–5).

chapter 6

Drawing Strength (Standing Postures)

As a Christian, your strength comes from the Lord. Psalm 46:1 calls Him "our refuge and strength." In Jeremiah 16:19, God is our "fortress." He is our power source, our firm foundation, and our rock.

His power is described as supreme (Ephesians 1:19–21), unlimited (Matthew 28:18), and everlasting (1 Timothy 6:16). He has the power to overcome Satan, forgive sins, perform miracles, and conquer all things.

Is there a machine at the gym that offers that kind of power? Is there a self-help book that can teach you to harness the willpower to do these things? Can you learn it, buy it, get it online? No. The only source for all this power comes from the Creator. And it's yours for the asking. "He gives power to those who are tired and worn out; he offers strength to the weak" (Isaiah 40:29). "For I can do everything with the help of Christ who gives me the strength I need" (Philippians 4:13).

Feeling God's power in your life happens when you admit your weakness. Rick Warren writes of finding God's power in our weakness in his best-selling book, *The Purpose Driven Life.* Given that we all have flaws, imperfections, and weaknesses, Warren writes that the more important issue is what we do with them. "Usually we deny our weaknesses, defend them, excuse them, hide them and resent them. This prevents God from using them the way He desires. God has a different perspective on your weaknesses. He says, 'My thoughts and my ways are higher than yours,' [Isaiah 55:9] so He often acts in ways that are the exact opposite of what we expect. We think that God only wants to use our strengths, but he also wants to use our weaknesses for His glory."[1]

He can use your weakness, and He can give you power. Once you admit you can't do it on your own, God can provide strength in any circumstance. You may begin to feel a confidence to speak God's truth in an uncertain setting. You may enjoy a reassuring peace when you encounter a tragedy. You may experience a boldness to turn from a lifestyle or behavior that is not pleasing to God.

Whatever the circumstance, God is the source of that strength. The help may not come in the form of an Old Testament miracle, but instead in the form of a caring friend, a wise pastor, or an unexpected opportunity for reflection. It may even come in the form of struggle, discomfort, or tragedy.

No matter the form, strength is a gift God provides His children. He simply wants you to feel His power and recognize the source. Failing to recognize God as the source of your power puts you back into a self-centered orbit, where everything revolves around you and your very limited capabilities.

With God as your power source, you have limitless capabilities. Nothing is outside the realm of possibility! With Him, you possess the power to move mountains, to effect change, and to be healed. So what are you waiting for? "Be strong with the Lord's mighty power" (Ephesians 6:10).

How Do I Feel God's Strength?

Take an inhale. There is power in that breath! Just as your breath fuels your body, God fuels your breath. He gave you life and sustains that life through the amazing and intricate respiratory process. With each inhale, you are literally breathing life into your body. You are allowing God's masterpiece to draw strength with each intake of oxygen. When you begin to recognize that power, establish it as the foundation for your postures, and then move in positions that demand more endurance, you are drawing strength.

Keep in mind that strength is established through resistance and endurance. You create resistance by moving into the heat-building postures and then develop endurance by holding those postures for several breaths and repeating those same postures over time. With repeated exposure, your body develops stamina and muscle memory so that it becomes less and less difficult to move through the postures.

Soon, your body begins to enjoy the strength postures as empowering and rejuvenating. You begin to struggle less and relax more. This release of your struggle, your expectations, and perceived limitations is the key to an effective and productive yoga practice. It is also the key to spiritual freedom in Christ.

Spiritual freedom is experienced when you stop struggling with your own limited strength, your personal agenda, and your perceived failures and you allow God to be the source of all your strength. "But the Lord stood with me and gave me strength" (2 Timothy 4:17). Letting go of your own sense of power allows God to unleash His mighty power in your life, a force far greater than anything we can imagine or that we could ever deserve.

Letting go is an opportunity for humility. The world tells us to be independent and self-sufficient, but God says the opposite. He tells the apostle Paul in 2 Corinthians 12:9, "My gracious favor is all you need. My power works best in your weakness." Give God an opportunity to work by admitting that you can't do it on your own. In that admission, that humility, that weakness, God can do amazing things.

Standing Postures

Standing postures are best included after a warm-up period and balance postures. With your muscles warm and your body aligned properly, you are ready to challenge your body with heat-building postures that develop strength and stamina. Again, make sure you are practicing at the level that is appropriate for you and how you are feeling today.

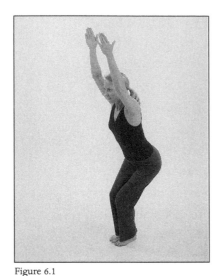

Figure 6.1

Chair—*strengthens and tones the feet, legs, hips, and buttocks; improves balance; tones the abs and back; stretches the calves* (figure 6.1)

1. Stand with your feet together. Try to spread your toes and set your feet firmly on the floor.

2. On your inhale, raise your arms overhead, bringing them shoulder-width apart with the palms facing in. Open your chest, and allow your shoulders to roll down your back.

3. On the exhale, draw the navel in toward the spine, flattening out the lower back.

4. Use the exhale to bend the knees, lowering the tailbone back and down as if sitting in an invisible chair.

5. Shift the majority of your weight onto your heels. Draw the shins and inner thighs in toward one another to keep the knees level and parallel and ankles strong. (A yoga block placed between the knees here is a good aid in keeping correct posture with the legs.)

6. Continue to lift the spine up and out through the crown of the head with arms extended.

7. Keep the face relaxed and belly firm.

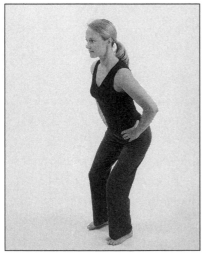

Figure 6.2

8. Keep your gaze forward and your neck in alignment with your spine.

9. Hold for five breaths.

High-intensity option
Continue drawing down in the legs and behind until the knees are bending toward 90 degrees.

Low-intensity option (figure 6.2)
Stand with feet hip-width apart instead of together, and lower your arms to rest gently at your hips.

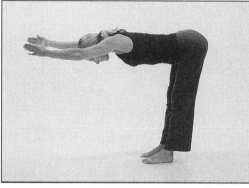

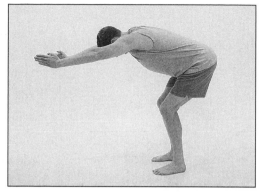

Figure 6.3

Figure 6.4

Strong Half Fold—*strengthens the legs, back, and abs; improves posture; builds heat* (figure 6.3)

1. From Mountain pose, use an inhale to raise the arms overhead and create as much length as you can up through the spine and out through the hands.

2. On the exhale, hinge from the hips as if you are folding into Forward Fold. But use your ab control to keep the body at a right angle to the legs, forming an L.

3. Keep the arms and crown of the head reaching outward, parallel to the floor.

4. Keep the feet grounded and the legs strong, pulling gently from the back of the knees.

5. Keep your gaze downward, letting the neck stay in alignment with the spine.

6. Pull back through the tailbone in the opposite direction as the arms are reaching.

7. Try not to round the back, but keep it flat, with the belly firm.

8. Soften the facial muscles as you stay here five breaths.

Low-intensity option (figure 6.4)

Keep the knees bent until your low back is flat and the belly is strong.

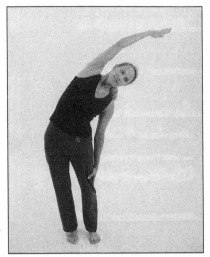

Figure 6.5

Side Lean—*lengthens the spine and side body, tones the legs, tones the belly, builds heat* (figure 6.5)

1. Stand in Mountain pose. On an inhale, raise the right arm up by the ear, palm facing in, to lengthen the entire right side of the body. Spread the fingers and energize out through the hand.

2. Use the exhale to firm the belly and relax the shoulders down the back.

3. Keeping the belly firm, the legs strong, and the chest and hips squared to the front of the room, lift up and over through the right arm, drawing it overhead and to the left to create a long arc.

4. Let the right hip lean slightly to the right as you complete the arc shape.

5. Both feet stay firm as you lean.

6. Keep your gaze forward and your face relaxed.

7. Stay here about five breaths before lifting up to standing on the inhale.

8. Use another exhale to complete the lean on the other side. Lean only as far as you can deeply breathe, can maintain control of your belly, and can feel comfortable through your back.

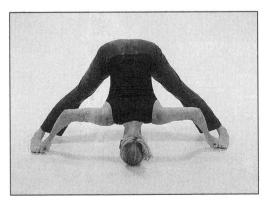

Figure 6.6

Standing Straddle Fold—*tones the legs, increases flexibility in hips and back, increases blood flow to the upper body and head, improves concentration, soothes the digestive system* (figure 6.6)

1. Turning sideways on your mat, step your feet four to four and a half feet apart.

2. Turn your heels out slightly so that the outside edges of your feet are lined up with the outside edges of your mat. Use both the inside and outside of your foot.

3. Relax your shoulders and keep your chest open.

4. Keep both hips level and squared toward the front of the room.

5. On an inhale, lift both arms overhead and lengthen the spine and neck.

6. On the exhale, hinge from the hips and fold toward the floor, reaching directly into the center of your legs.

7. On the next inhale, reach for your toes with each hand, holding the big toe with the pointer finger. (It's OK if you aren't able to reach your toes just yet. In this case, grab the calf and use it as resistance.)

8. Pull gently against the toes (or calves), flatten your spine, pull your chest forward, and glance halfway up.

9. Keep your legs as straight as possible and hips level.

10. Keeping the spine long and flat, use your next exhale to fold downward again, bringing the crown of the head toward the floor. The elbows will need to bend upward to create space for you to fold down. Think about trying to create a right angle with the upper arm and forearm.

11. Keep your belly firm, legs strong, and both the inside and outside of the foot engaged.

12. Stay here for five breaths, with your face and neck relaxed.

Low-intensity option (figure 6.7)

1. If the forward bend is difficult with straight legs, simply bend your knees slightly to release pressure in the lower back.

2. You may also choose to perform this pose without grabbing your toes, but instead resting the hands on the floor between the feet. *If you have high blood pressure, be careful, because this is considered an inversion and may be dangerous for you.*

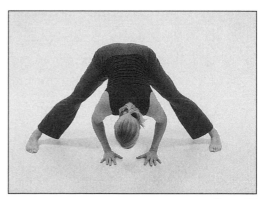

Figure 6.7

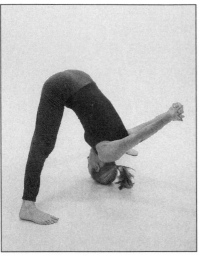

Figure 6.8

Standing Straddle with Arms Overhead—*same as the previous pose but also encourages a greater flexibility in the shoulders and upper back* (figure 6.8)

1. On an inhale, roll back up to standing with the legs still four to four-and-a-half feet apart.

2. Relax the shoulders down the back on the exhale.

3. On your next inhale, lift the arms to outstretched at shoulder level, lifting your spine and neck, opening the chest, and energizing out through all ten fingertips.

4. On the exhale, interlock your fingers behind your back. Keep your arms straight, but try not to lock your elbows.

5. On the inhale, lift your chest, engage your abs. Press your hands away from your back. If it is difficult for you to keep your hands interlocked, grab a strap, a towel, or a sock to hold between the hands.

6. Use your exhale to fold forward, bringing the crown of the head toward the floor directly between your feet.

7. Relax your shoulders and your face, and let your arms fall farther overhead with each exhale. You should find a little movement with each breath. Think about creating space up and out of the legs on each inhale, then folding and drawing the arms over on each exhale.

8. Stay here at least five breaths before using an inhale to lift back up to standing.

Low-intensity option
As in the previous pose, you may choose to bend your knees slightly.

Standing Straddle with Twist—*same as straddle fold but also integrates the twist which wrings out old blood and fluids from the abs, making room for freshly oxygenated, nutrient-rich blood; also strengthens neck and obliques* (figure 6.9)

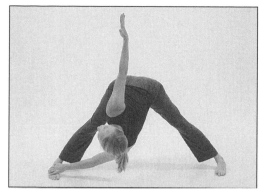

Figure 6.9

1. Stay in the wide straddle position, with both feet engaged and legs strong.

2. Keep the spine long, the belly firm, and the face relaxed.

3. On an inhale, reach the arms overhead to create length.

4. Use your exhale to hinge at the hips and fold toward the floor with a flat back. Let your hands rest on the floor between your feet.

5. Look toward your right foot and bring your left hand across to grab the toe or right above the ankle (and remember our rule of never grabbing on the joint).

6. Turn and reach for the sky with your right hand, drawing back with the right shoulder and extending up with the fingertips.

7. Allow the neck to follow the right hand to gaze upward, extending through the crown of the head.

8. Use the inhale to lengthen the spine and draw your left elbow toward the floor.

9. Use the exhale to twist farther toward the right foot, without changing the direction of your hips. Keep the hips level and squared toward the floor.

10. Keep the belly firm and the face relaxed.

11. Stay here for five breaths before releasing and following the same sequence on the other side.

High-intensity option (figure 6.10)

After using the extended arm to reach for the sky, turn the palm around and wrap the arm around behind the back for additional twist.

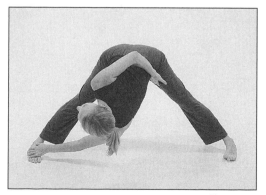

Figure 6.10

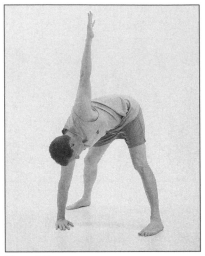

Figure 6.11

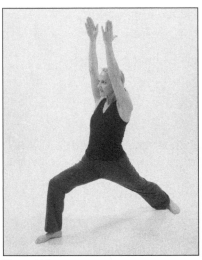

Figure 6.12

Low-intensity option (figure 6.11)

1. Rather than looking up with your twist, keep your neck relaxed and gaze downward toward the floor.

2. You may also choose not to reach for the toe, but instead to place the reaching hand on the floor between the midpoint of the legs and the foot.

Warrior I—*strengthens and tones the legs, brings flexibility to the hips, improves posture, strengthens the back* (figure 6.12)

1. From the Standing Straddle, turn your right foot to face the front of the room, toes and knees pointing in the same direction.

2. Let your hips follow the turn of the foot to face forward.

3. Turn the left heel out away from the body to create a 45- to 60-degree angle. If you looked back from right heel to left foot, the right heel and the left arch would be lined up front to back.

4. From this strong stance, bend the right knee to 90 degrees, creating a right angle with the thigh and shin. The knee should rest directly over the heel. The left leg stays straight and strong, with energy directed to both the inside and the outside of the foot.

5. On an inhale, bring your arms overhead, drawing them in toward your ears with palms facing inward. Keep the shoulders relaxed, but engage all the way up the arms with fingers spread and reaching.

6. Continue to work on squaring your hips forward, drawing the left hip forward and right hip back.

7. With your balance and weight centering front to back, begin to think about the weight drawing up. Start from the hips and lift from the spine, the sternum, the heart, the neck, and the arms.

8. Keep your gaze forward as you firm the belly, letting the hips tuck, the lower back fill out, and the tailbone point down instead of back.

9. Don't push your chest and ribs forward. That could cause compression in the mid- and low spine. Instead, keep the spine long and lifting.

10. Keep the front knee deeply bent and the weight distributed evenly between the inside and outside of the foot.

11. Stay here for five breaths before straightening the leg, turning back to Standing Straddle, then turning the left foot out to begin the posture on the other side.

Low-intensity option
Create a shorter stance by bringing the legs a little closer together and bend the knee to a more comfortable position.

Visualization suggestion
As you stand in strong Warrior I pose, feel empowerment through the Holy Spirit on each energizing inhale. On the exhale, let every burden release out of the body through the fingertips as you reach upward toward heaven. Name those burdens and release them to God one by one on each relaxing out-breath.

Warrior II—*tones and strengthens the legs, opens the hips, strengthens the foot and ankle, improves balance and posture* (figure 6.13)

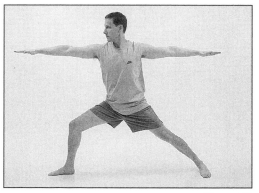

Figure 6.13

1. From Warrior I, reach your spine tall on an inhale and then use your exhale to turn your chest and hips open back to the center of your legs.

2. Let your arms float down until they are outstretched and activated in a T position parallel to the floor, with palms facing down.

3. Make sure that your front knee has remained deeply bent and toes grounded. Keep the knee centered over the foot, with both the inside and outside of the foot engaged.

4. Notice that the back leg has remained straight and strong, with the foot at a 45- to 60-degree angle.

5. Use another exhale to bend your front knee closer to that 90-degree angle.

6. Lift out of the hips and up through the spine and neck, keeping the face relaxed.

7. At the same time, drop your shoulders down your back and pull in opposite directions with the arms, fingers spread and engaged fully.

8. Keep your belly firm and lifting, drawing the navel toward the spine to create the hip tuck that will ultimately protect the lower back.

9. Keep your gaze concentrated over the front fingertips.

10. Stay here five breaths before moving to the other leg.

Low-intensity option

As in Warrior I, shorten the stance of your legs and keep the knee bent only as low as is comfortable.

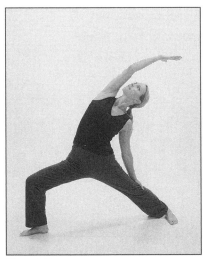

Figure 6.14

Reverse Warrior—*creates an opening through the chest, neck, and side body; strengthens the leg, ankles, back, and arms; improves posture and hip flexibility* (figure 6.14)

1. From Warrior II, lengthen up through both sides of the body on the inhale.

2. Relax the shoulders down the back on the exhale.

3. On the next inhale, turn the front palm up and reach for the sky. Let the front body open as you reach.

4. Let the back hand drop back and rest comfortably on the back of the thigh. Be careful not to push on the knee or rest too much weight on the leg.

5. As the front body lengthens, continue opening back to gently arc the back.

6. Let your gaze follow the hand as it reaches up and back.

7. Keep the face relaxed and the belly firm.

8. Take five breaths here before moving to the other side.

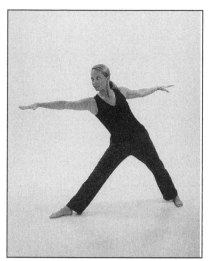

Figure 6.15a

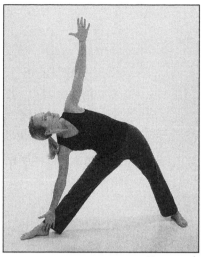

Figure 6.15b

Triangle—*creates openness through the chest and back; strengthens the leg, ankles, back, arms, and arches; lengthens the torso, side body, and hamstrings; improves posture and hip flexibility; stimulates the kidneys and digestive system (figures 6.15a and 6.15b)*

1. From Standing Straddle, again turn your right foot forward to the front of the room.

2. Keep the hips and chest open as in Warrior II, while you adjust the left heel out to a 45- to 60-degree angle. Keep both legs strong and straight, using both sides of the feet, inside and outside.

3. On your inhale, lift the arms parallel to the floor, with palms facing down. Reach through the fingertips, opening the chest and releasing the shoulders to float down the back on the exhale.

4. Look out over the right hand.

5. Keep the chest open, the spine long, and belly firm as you use the next inhale to reach the right hand and torso out as if you are trying to extend beyond the right foot (figure 6.15a).

6. After reaching out as far as you can, use the exhale to lower the right hand down to the shin or foot. Remember that where your hand falls on your leg is not nearly as important as having the correct posture through the back and hips.

7. Reach through the left hand as you attempt to get your body completely stacked in a frontal plane. Your arms should be stacked in one vertical line, with minimal weight resting in the left hand. Instead, lift out of the left hand as you create length and openness toward the right (figure 6.15b).

8. Open your chest, lining the right shoulder directly under the left.

9. Draw the right hip forward and the left hip back to line them up squared to the front of the room.

10. Keep the belly firm, with the tailbone scooped under to breathe into the lower back.

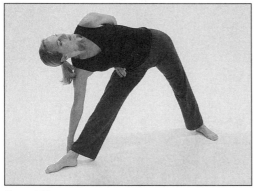
Figure 6.16

11. Turn your face to look up toward the extended hand and hold for five deep breaths.

High-intensity option (figure 6.16)

1. From Triangle pose, attempt to turn the left palm around and drop the arm behind the back, reaching for the thigh. This will facilitate further opening through the chest and shoulders.

2. You may also choose to place your hand on the floor on the outside of the foot for further challenge. Remember to drop the hand only as far as you can maintain that frontal plane.

Low-intensity option (figure 6.17)

1. If you are unable to keep the body stacked, move the hand further up the shin or onto the thigh. This is also a great opportunity to use a block, placed directly under the hand for support.

2. You may also choose to release the neck, allowing your gaze to fall downward to the floor, if the neck feels stressed or overtired.

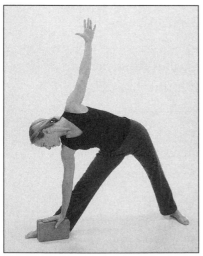
Figure 6.17

Reverse Triangle—*wrings toxins out of the body, facilitates digestive function, relieves lower back pain, improves balance, strengthens legs and neck, improves hip flexibility* (figures 6.18a and 6.18b)

1. From Triangle pose, keep your feet in the same position but bring your hands to rest gently at your hips.

2. Take as much time as you need to direct your hips to face over the front leg (start with the right in front). Try to square your hips over the leg, with the spine and neck long (figure 6.18a).

3. As the elbows point out, let them serve as directional reminders for the hips.

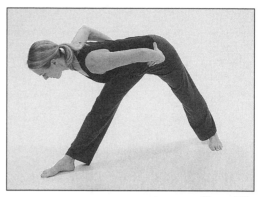

Figure 6.18a

4. Firm the belly and fully engage both legs.

5. Without changing the direction of the hips, drop your left hand to rest on the floor on the inside of your foot. If you don't feel comfortable reaching that far, drop your hand to your right shin, foot, or rest it on your block. Make sure you are stable using your firm belly and strong legs.

6. On an inhale, draw your right arm up and out toward the sky.

7. Press through both arms to create a long vertical line.

8. As you create this rotation, pull your right hip back and your left hip forward. Let the entire torso twist at a level that is challenging yet comfortable.

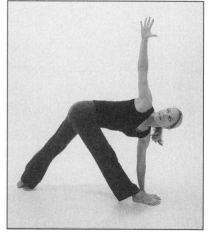

Figure 6.18b

9. Relax the shoulders down the back.

10. Soften your face, turn your head, and gaze toward the extended hand (figure 6.18b).

11. Think about lengthening the spine and neck with each inhale.

12. Continue with your rotation on the exhale.

13. Stay here about five breaths before you exhale the hand down and inhale the upper body back up to standing.

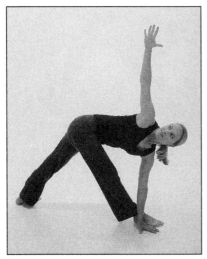

Figure 6.19

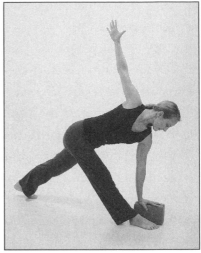

Figure 6.20

High-intensity option (figure 6.19)

Try to rest your hand on the outside of the foot for additional rotation.

Low-intensity option (figure 6.20)

1. Use a block for support, positioned on the inside of the foot. If you have trouble balancing, place the block at a greater distance away from the foot.

2. If rotating your hips is challenging, you may lift your back heel slightly off the floor to allow less resistance from the legs.

3. As always, if the neck is sensitive, allow your gaze to fall downward toward the floor.

Side Angle—*stretches the entire side of the body, provides strength and stability for the legs, trims the waist and hips, improves respiratory function, relieves back pain, cultivates balance and coordination* (figure 6.21)

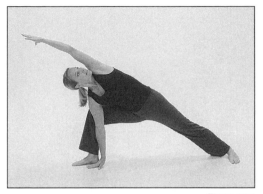

Figure 6.21

1. From Standing Straddle, point the right toes toward the front of the room at a right angle from the left foot. Make sure the knee and toes are facing the same direction. Keep your hips and shoulders squared to the center of the legs.

2. On an inhale, bring the arms out to shoulder height. Engage the arms out in both directions, reaching through the fingertips. Keep the shoulders relaxed and drawing down the back.

3. On an exhale, fully engage the abs and bend the right knee so that the thigh and calf form a right angle with each other (as in Warrior II). Keep your left leg straight and extended, drawing through both the inside and outside of the foot.

4. Use another inhale to ensure the spine and neck are long.

5. On the next exhale, slowly drop your right hand down to rest on the inside of the foot. Try to place your entire palm down on the floor or block (you may need to start with your fingertips first).

6. On the next inhale, draw your left shoulder back, open your chest, and look toward the ceiling. Try to get your body as two dimensional as possible.

7. On the exhale, stretch your left arm up and over the head until it creates a long diagonal line with the rest of your body. Turn the left palm to face down. Let your chin draw close to the upper arm as you look toward the sky.

8. Continue to use each inhale to lengthen and each exhale to tuck your tailbone under with the belly firm.

9. Stay here for five breaths before straightening the leg back up to Standing Straddle on an inhale.

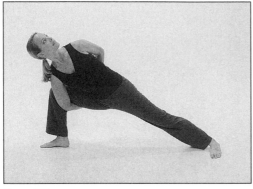

Figure 6.22

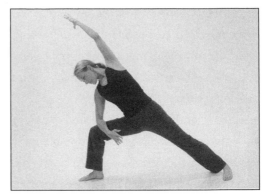

Figure 6.23

High-intensity option (figure 6.22)

1. Instead of placing your hand on the inside of the foot, try placing it on the outside for further challenge.

2. You may choose to bind your arms behind you by bringing the left hand behind your back and reaching through the legs with your right until they connect.

3. Remember, it is more important to create the proper alignment than it is to add intensity. Make sure you are still upright, as if sandwiched between two panes of glass.

Low-intensity option (figure 6.23)

1. Instead of reaching for the floor, place your elbow on the knee, while keeping the knee bent.

2. If your neck is sensitive or stiff, let your gaze face forward or downward.

Crescent—*creates strength in the legs, improves posture and coordination in the body, lengthens the spine, improves focus* (figure 6.24)

1. From Standing Straddle position, move into Lunge by turning both feet to face the right, creating a straight line between the feet.

2. Press back through the left heel and bend the right knee until the right knee is resting over the right heel (never let the knee push out past the toes).

3. Rest your hands on the floor (or on two blocks) on either side of the feet. Square your hips to face downward.

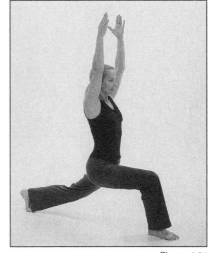

Figure 6.24

4. Firm your belly, tucking your tailbone under.

5. On an inhale, sweep your arms up along with your spine until you are standing tall from the hips to the crown of the head.

6. Let the arms energize upward through the fingertips, while the shoulders rest down the back.

7. Engage both legs by pressing through the balls of the feet. Keep the back leg straight and strong by lifting the quadricep and the knee.

8. Continue to let the hips face the front of the room and the tailbone point downward.

9. As your gaze is concentrated forward, use each inhale to lengthen up and out of the spine and use each exhale to sink gently down into hips and legs.

10. Keep your face relaxed as you remain in this pose for five breaths.

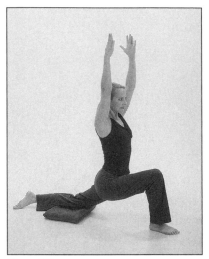

Figure 6.25

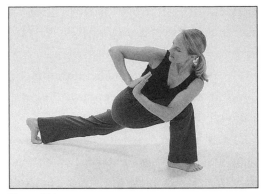

Figure 6.26

Low-intensity option (figure 6.25)

1. Instead of creating a straight line between your feet, move the back foot out about three to four inches to the side to make it easier to balance.

2. If you are still struggling in this pose, consider dropping the back knee to the mat. If you drop the knee, make sure that it is still lengthened back at a long angle rather than resting under the hips.

3. Be sure to fold up the end of the mat or use a towel under the knee for extra cushion, if your knees are sensitive.

Revolving Crescent (Prayer Hands)—*wrings out toxins, strengthens the back and legs, opens the chest, and creates flexibility up and down the spine* (figure 6.26)

1. From Crescent, use an inhale to lengthen up as preparation for the twist.

2. On the exhale, bring your hands together and rest them down toward your heart in prayer position.

3. Turn and look out over the right side, allowing the entire torso to turn with you.

4. Keep the legs engaged and belly firm.

5. Use an inhale to lengthen one more time while in this rotation.

6. Then use the exhale to drop the left elbow to outside of the right knee, using it as resistance to facilitate the full twist. Keep your hands pressing together in

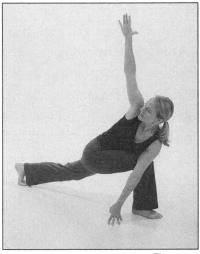

Figure 6.27

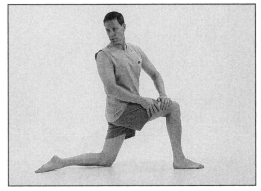

Figure 6.28

prayer, so that the elbows are wide. With the left elbow on the inside of the right knee, the right elbow is pointing up toward the sky.

7. Let your gaze follow that elbow.

8. Continue to lengthen the torso on each inhale and further the rotation on the exhale.

9. Keep your navel drawn in toward your spine and your right shoulder drawing back.

10. Stay in this twist for five breaths.

High-intensity option (figure 6.27)

If you are able to twist with your elbow fully on the outside of the knee, then you may consider further challenge by bringing your lower hand to the floor on the outside of your right leg and reaching your upper hand toward the sky.

Low-intensity option (figure 6.28)

1. As you may have chosen to do in Crescent, you can drop the back knee gently to the floor at a long angle away from the hips.

2. If you are unable to reach your elbow across the knee, simply place both hands on the right thigh to use as resistance to create the twist.

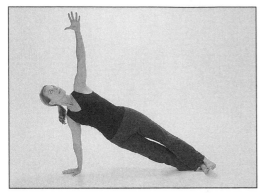

Figure 6.29

Side Plank—*tones the arms and strengthens the shoulder, tones the abs and midsection, improves focus and coordination* (figure 6.29)

1. From Plank or Tabletop, straighten the legs and bring your feet together so that the inner thighs and shins are drawing in toward one another.

2. Spin your feet to the left, with one foot stacked atop the other (or crossed at the ankles, if you find it difficult to balance).

3. Bring your left hand up to reach for the sky. Your right hand should be directly under the right shoulder, creating a long line from hand to hand.

4. Stack the upper hip directly over the lower one to align your body in a frontal plane, with the tailbone pointed down toward the feet.

5. Engage all the muscles of your body in an effort to keep weight balanced and lifting out of the right shoulder. Let the power for this lift start with the firm belly and move outward to the extremities.

6. Let your shoulders drop down the back as you create space.

7. Relax your face and turn your gaze upward toward the extended hand, if possible.

8. Stay here for three to five breaths—or less, if you feel too much weight coming into the right shoulder.

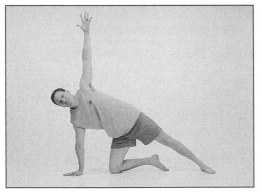

Figure 6.30

Low-intensity option (figure 6.30)

If you know that you have shoulder issues, do not try the full posture for Side Plank. Instead, there is a healthier option for you that still requires strength and balance but doesn't put nearly the same amount of pressure on your shoulders.

1. Rather than straightening both legs, simply drop the right knee to the floor directly

under the right hip and spin your left leg open by grabbing the floor with the inside of the left foot.

2. Make sure that you have created a straight line with the right hand, right knee, and left foot.

3. Remember to cushion the knee on the floor if it is sensitive.

Indian Squat—*stretches the muscles around the knees, lubricates the knee joint, creates flexibility in the hip, improves posture and balance* (figure 6.31)

1. From Mountain pose, separate the feet to the outer edges of your mat, with the toes turning out to the corners of the room.

2. On an inhale, lift the arms to reach overhead, creating a long spine and neck.

3. On the exhale, bring the hands together and draw the arms down to your heart.

4. As you are drawing the hands down, let the knees bend and let your tailbone drop down between the legs.

5. Keep the belly firm as you lower the body between the knees.

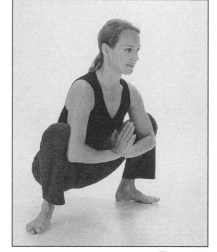

Figure 6.31

6. Notice that the knees stay up and the feet stay firmly resting on the floor.

7. Once you've lowered to your lowest point, let your elbows rest on the inside of the knees for additional resistance.

8. Keep the spine and neck lifting and face relaxed.

9. Stay here for five or more breaths as you let the muscles around the knees stretch. Listen carefully to those knees as you are breathing.

Low-intensity option
Lower only as far as your knees feel comfortable.

Prayer for Strength

"Let your roots grow down into him and draw up nourishment from him, so you will grow in faith, strong and vigorous in the truth you were taught. Let your lives overflow with thanksgiving for all he has done" (Colossians 2:7).

Removing Barriers (Floor Postures)

GOD DESIRES TO DRAW NEAR TO YOU. HE PROMISES IN SCRIPTURE THAT IF WE DRAW near to Him, He will draw near to us (James 4:8). How do you draw near to God? You remove the barriers that create separation.

Sometimes your barriers might be practical ones, such as time or physical discomfort. You simply don't feel like meeting with God because your body is weary, hurting, and generally uncomfortable. Your physical symptoms literally create a barrier to realizing the joy, peace, and comfort that come from your relationship with Christ.

Other times, emotional and psychological barriers create a gulf of separation from God. Our will, our wounds, and our struggles seem far more important at the moment than what God has to offer.

But if you learn to look at every experience through God's eyes, Scripture promises:

o *When you turn over your will, you receive His guidance and direction.* "I will instruct you and teach you in the way you should go; I will counsel you and watch over you" (Psalm 32:8 NIV).

o *When you turn over your wounds, you receive wholeness and joy.* "That is why we never give up. Though our bodies are dying, our spirits are being renewed every day. For our present troubles are quite small and won't last very long. Yet they produce for us an immeasurably great glory that will last forever! So we don't look at the troubles we see right now; rather, we look forward to what we have not yet seen. For the troubles we see now will soon be over, but the joys to come will last forever" (2 Corinthians 4:16–18).

o *When you let God use your struggles, you experience spiritual growth, depth of Christian character, and a readiness to be used for what God desires.* "Whenever trouble comes your way, let it be an opportunity for joy. For when your faith is tested, your endurance has a chance to grow. So let it grow, for when your endurance is fully developed, you will be strong in character and ready for anything" (James 1:2–4).

The best exercise program for our underdeveloped character muscles is struggle—the very thing we try to avoid and pray never happens to us. Yet the Bible tells us that hardship provides lessons that bring depth to our lives. If we don't struggle, we have no chance to flex those muscles; as a result, they atrophy. Letting God have not only your blessings but also your hurts brings wholeness and perspective to your life. You let God use your struggles, in part, by how you react to difficult situations.

It has been said that life consists of 10 percent what has happened to you and 90 percent of what you learned from it. You become the compilation, not of your circumstances, but of your reaction to your circumstances. Who do you want to be: a representative of anger and frustration, or a depiction of God-given joy and peace?

Making that pivotal change in your perspective comes from learning to look at every struggle through God's eyes, filtered through His heart of unconditional love. Consider every difficult circumstance as an opportunity for growth in Christ, as an opportunity to be readied for His assignments, to be strengthened in your faith.

Examine your life and the biggest hurts you have experienced. Expand your memory of those experiences to include not only the hurt, but also how God may have used those experiences. Reflect on how you and those around you were changed by the events. If you can't see God working in those struggles, consider what barriers might need to be removed to bridge the gap between your struggle and God's hand.

React with Surrender

What should be your reaction to struggles? Total surrender to God. When you react with deference to God's will, then you are effectively removing the barriers that keep you separated from Him. You are indicating that you are willing and available for God to shape you and guide you toward a life of fruitfulness, joyfulness, and contentment. You begin to experience the ultimate freedom that comes only from living a life submitted to Him.

A great example of surrender came as Greg and I recently celebrated our fifteenth wedding anniversary with a trip to Costa Rica. We stayed at a yoga spa, which offered a variety of yoga classes during the week, from advanced to restorative. Greg, being the wonderful husband that he is, planned the trip, although he really struggles to enjoy the yoga experience. When we practice at home, he works hard to make the pose happen, even if his body is resisting, which usually results in a labored (or nonexistent) breath and a very pained expression.

But we attended a class together in Costa Rica in which the instructor told Greg exactly what he needed to hear to understand and fully enjoy the benefits of the practice. As Greg lay there struggling, our instructor asked, "Do you like sports?" Greg responded an enthusiastic "Yes!" (Now we were talking his language.) The instructor explained, "In sports, you *do*. In yoga, you *let go*."

Ahh, you could see the tension release from my struggling husband's body and face. He had been given permission to let go and find contentment with where he was. His pose didn't have to look like my pose or the instructor's pose. He was free to enjoy the benefit of the posture from where he was right then. No more struggle, no more fighting what his body wanted to do. He could let his breath work and accept the response. He reacted with a surrender that I had not seen in his practice before.

That is what God asks of you. You will experience struggle. You are guaranteed hardship. But if you respond with a graceful surrender, God will reward you with a contentment that leads to freedom. You become free from the pressure to have it all, to be the best, to never fail. Jesus tells us in Matthew 11:28–30: "Come to me, all of you who are weary and carry heavy burdens, and I will give you rest. Take my yoke upon you. Let me teach you, because I am humble and gentle, and you will find rest for your souls. For my yoke fits perfectly, and the burden I give you is light."

Outstretched to Freedom

Taking the same perspective with your body's struggles will provide you with a comfort and freedom you may have never experienced. It is a comfort that comes from creating space, heat, and ultimately flexibility throughout your muscles. It is achieved by attempting floor postures that challenge your flexibility (struggle), and then submitting to the breath to find movement in that pose (surrender).

There is no ultimate goal, such as reaching your toes or putting your foot behind your head. You are simply moving toward greater and greater freedom from your physical barriers by challenging your muscles toward greater flexibility and creating greater range of motion.

You will never experience any lasting growth from forcing or coercing your body to change. Instead, the result will more likely be frustration, pain, or (worst case) an injury. To safeguard against those undesirable consequences, you must choose to submit to the pose by creating a body awareness that tells you how far you should go and then surrendering fully to the breath for deeper movement into the posture. Over time, you will be amazed at the growth you will experience from simply letting go.

As you begin to develop more flexibility through your floor postures, first notice what your body is saying in the struggle. Next, evaluate what your response is to your body. Are you forcing or surrendering? Are you relaxing or tensing? What does your body/mind/heart do when you "hit the wall"? Reflect on James 1:2–4 for your appropriate response.

Transition to floor postures after you have completed adequate warm-up, balance to realign, and standing postures to build additional heat. Move directly from heat-building to floor so that you can use the heat to create more movement in your stretches. Keep the breath flowing deeply in the balanced complete breath outlined in chapter 3. Also, remember your general posture cues for proper sitting. Keep your blanket handy in case you need to support your knees in kneeling or your buttocks in sitting.

Seated Floor Postures

If your sitting bones tend to lift off the floor or if you are uncomfortable in any of the sitting postures, try using a folded blanket under the buttocks to elevate your hips and provide added cushion.

Staff—*prepares the body for more rigorous seated postures, lengthens the spine, stretches the legs* (figure 7.1)

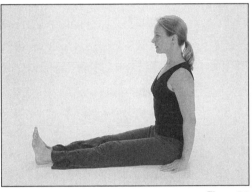

Figure 7.1

1. Start your seated postures here to properly align your body. Sit on the floor and stretch your legs out in front of you.
2. Keep your feet together with toes and knees pointed toward the ceiling.
3. Place your hands flat on the floor on either side of your buttocks, with your fingers facing forward and your palms gently pressing down into the floor.
4. Engage your thigh muscles and push out through the ball of the foot. (You know you're pushing through the ball when the toes spread.)
5. Lift your chest and relax the shoulders down the back.
6. Lengthen the spine by pulling from the base of the spine up through the crown of the head.
7. Keep your legs as straight as possible, but don't lock the knees.

8. Draw your navel in toward the spine to engage your abs and protect your lower back.

9 Keep your eyes focused straight ahead.

10. Stay here for at least five deep breaths.

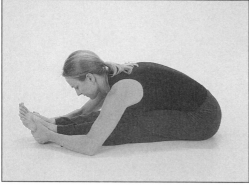

Figure 7.2

Seated Forward Bend—*awakens the spine, stimulates the nerves at the base of the spine, stretches the hamstrings, increases flexibility in the spine and hips* (figure 7.2)

1. Start in Staff pose, with your legs extended in front of you and the spine tall.

2. On an inhale, reach the arms overhead, lengthening from the hips to the hands.

3. Exhale and hinge from the hips to fold forward. Lead from your chest, with your back remaining flat instead of rounding.

4. Reach for the legs or feet, depending on where along the legs you are able to grab. (Remember, we never grab right on a joint, so avoid holding at the knees or ankles.)

5. Keep your legs as straight as possible and your abs engaged by drawing the navel in and up.

6. To ensure that you are moving outward toward your toes and not just downward, take the next inhale and glance up, pulling the chest forward and lengthening the spine farther over the legs.

7. On the exhale, sink back down toward the legs with the spine as long as it will go and the legs as straight as possible.

8. Point the chin down toward the knees with the face relaxed.

9. Stay here for five or more breaths. Notice how each exhale allows you a little more movement downward toward your legs and outward toward your toes. Remember, the goal is not necessarily to reach your toes, but to release in the posture smoothly, without forcing or straining your body.

Low-intensity option (figure 7.3)

1. If you are having trouble reaching out-ward, grab a strap (or use a towel, scarf, or tie) and wrap it around the bottoms of the feet.

2. Bend the knees and hold the ends of the strap with your hands.

3. Gently pull on your strap as you exhale, and continue lowering downward.

4. If your back feels particularly stiff, try not reaching for the toes at all but instead bending the knees and wrapping the arms around the legs to draw the chest close.

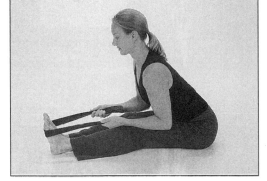

Figure 7.3

Bent Knee Seated Forward Fold—*relieves backache, loosens hamstrings, encourages flexibility in hips and spine* (figure 7.4)

1. This fold is a little less intense than the previous one but provides very similar benefits. Start again in Staff pose with both legs extended.

2. Bend the right knee and tuck the heel of the right foot into your groin, letting the sole of the foot press into the inner thigh of the left leg.

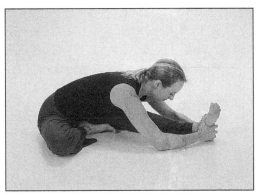

Figure 7.4

3. Relax the right knee open, letting it fall close to the floor.

4. Engage the muscles of the left leg and draw your abdominal muscles in and up.

5. On an inhale, reach your arms overhead, lengthening from hip to hands.

6. On the exhale, hinge at the hips and fold forward over the left leg, reaching to grasp the left leg or foot. Keep your shoulders level and your weight resting directly over the left leg. Concentrate on maintaining the alignment between your forehead and the extended leg.

7. Keep your spine as straight and long as possible and your leg as straight as possible.

8. To encourage lengthening of the spine, use an inhale to glance up, drawing your chest forward and drawing your body longer down the extended leg.

9. On the exhale, relax and fold to your deepest position without compromising the length of your back.

10. Relax your face and breathe deeply for five or more breaths, noticing that you have a little more movement downward and outward with each exhale.

11. On an inhale, return to an upright position.

12. Release the bent leg on an exhale, and begin the posture on the other side.

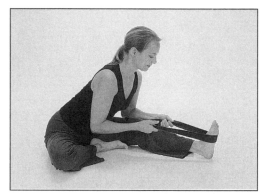

Figure 7.5

Low-intensity option (figure 7.5)

1. The use of a strap around the extended foot will aid in the lengthening process and create proper alignment.

2. If necessary, you may also bend the extended leg slightly to allow for more work in the back by relieving some of the stretch for the leg.

Seated Spinal Twist—*reduces stiffness in the back and neck; realigns the vertebrae; strengthens the neck; opens the shoulders, chest, and hips; massages the abs; aids in elimination, stimulates the thyroid* (Remember, twists are usually not suitable during pregnancy.) (figure 7.6)

1. Start in Staff pose, with legs extended and spine long.

2. Keep your shoulders open and relaxed.

3. Bend your right knee, and draw that knee in toward the chest to allow it to step over the left leg.

4. Place the sole of your right foot on the outside of your left knee. Maintain a long extension of the spine and extended leg.

5. Use your left arm to wrap around the bent right knee, drawing it close to the chest.

6. Place your right hand on the floor by your hip or buttocks. Let that hand help create proper lengthening in the spine.

7. On an inhale, press through the right palm while extending up through the crown of the head.

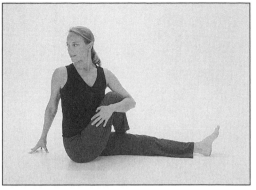

Figure 7.6

8. On the exhale, engage your abs and rotate your upper body slowly to the right. Keep your right foot firmly resting on the floor.

9. Let your gaze follow this rotation until you are looking over the right shoulder. Continue this rotating movement with each breath.

10. Hold for five or more breaths, with face relaxed and chest open, before moving to the other side.

High-intensity option (figure 7.7)

1. If you feel comfortable with the rotating movement of the spine, try bringing the right foot back to the inside of the left leg. Place the sole of the foot firmly on the floor close to the buttocks.

2. This time when you begin the rotation, use the elbow on the outside of the right leg to create resistance to keep the knee close to the chest and keep the spine rotating fully.

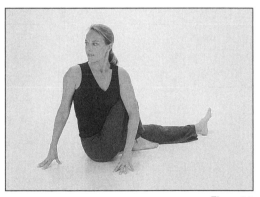

Figure 7.7

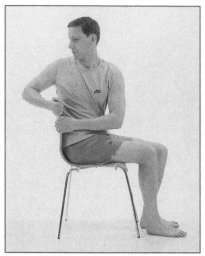

Figure 7.8

Low-intensity option (figure 7.8)

1. If you have tight hips or knee problems, try doing this position while seated in a chair. With both feet resting firmly on the floor, chest and hips facing forward, engage the abs and lengthen the spine.

2. Reach around to the right side of your chair (or the back of the chair if you can reach it) with both hands. Pull gently against the chair to create rotation through the spine.

3. Let your gaze follow this rotation. Hold for five breaths before moving to the other side.

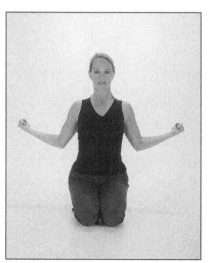

Figure 7.9

Blade—*opens the chest, improves posture, strengthens the rhomboid muscle, strengthens the biceps* (figure 7.9)

1. From Staff pose, cross your legs comfortably or tuck them behind you until the buttocks is resting on the heels.

2. Lengthen from the base of the spine upward to the crown of the head.

3. Relax the face and engage the abs, creating a tuck of the tailbone.

4. On an inhale, raise the arms outstretched at the side, with palms facing up.

5. On an exhale, make a medium-intensity fist with both hands, bend the elbows, and draw them in toward the back of the ribcage.

6. On each inhale, continue to lengthen upward through the neck and spine.

7. On each exhale, continue to draw the elbows in and back to open the chest. Let the shoulder blades pull together.

8. Stay here for about five breaths before inhaling the arms back out straight and then relaxing them to your sides on an exhale.

Butterfly—*improves posture; stretches inner thighs, groin, and hips; eases lower back pain; increases flexibility of knees; encourages blood flow to the pelvis, abs, and back; helps women maintain a healthy menstrual cycle; useful during pregnancy as it helps the body prepare for childbirth* (figure 7.10)

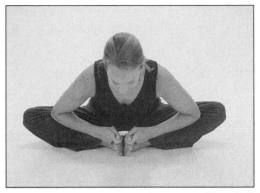

Figure 7.10

1. From Staff pose, bring the soles of your feet together, letting your knees drop comfortably to the sides.

2. Grip your feet and gently draw your heels back closer to the groin.

3. Inhale and lengthen your spine and neck, pulling up through the crown of the head. Open your chest.

4. On an exhale, roll your shoulders down and away from your ears. Stay here a couple of breaths as you use each exhale to relax your shoulders down and relax your hips open so that your knees move down toward the floor.

5. On your next inhale, lengthen up through the spine and lift your chest.

6. On the next exhale, hinge from the hips and fold forward from the lower back. Do not round the back or hunch your shoulders. How far forward you lean is not nearly as important as maintaining the correct posture.

7. As you relax on each exhale, let your chin rest downward toward the floor ahead of your feet. Only fold as far as you feel comfortable, resting the knees open and the chest downward with each exhale.

8. Stay here for at least five breaths.

High-intensity option (figure 7.11)

1. As you are able to relax downward, move your hands away from your feet and try dropping your elbows to the floor.

2. After a few breaths, if you feel you have more movement, slide your elbows out and try laying your forehead on the floor

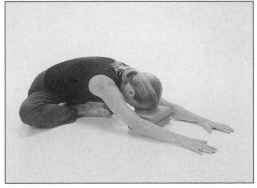

Figure 7.11

(or on a block, rolled up towel, or stacked fists). Allowing the forehead a place to relax will help in letting the hips and back release as well.

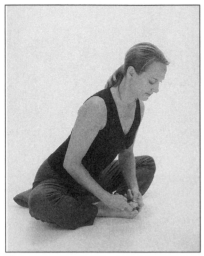

Figure 7.12

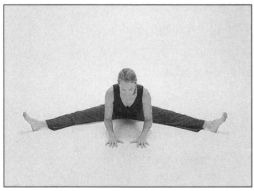

Figure 7.13

Low-intensity option (figure 7.12)

1. Sitting on a blanket, which will slightly elevate your hips, may provide some added comfort.

2. Also, if your hips are very tight and will not relax downward, forget about the lean entirely and stay with relaxing the hips alone.

Straddle Forward Fold—*opens the hips and sacrum, encourages blood flow to the pelvis, can alleviate menstrual pain, stretches the inner thigh and spine* (figure 7.13)

1. Sit with your legs stretched out in front of you. Notice that your spine is tall and your shoulders relaxed and down away from your ears.

2. Keep your chest strong and your face relaxed.

3. Separate your legs one at a time a comfortable distance apart.

4. Gently press the back of the legs into the floor so that your toes and knees point upward toward the ceiling.

5. Draw your hips forward, with your sitting bones squarely on the floor.

6. Place both hands on the floor between your legs, with palms facing down and elbows soft. Inhale, lifting your chest and lengthening your spine and neck.

7. Exhale and fold forward, being careful not to round the back or bring your sitting bones off the floor. On each inhale, continue to lengthen and draw the chest outward. On each exhale, continue to bring your chin and chest farther toward the floor as you walk your hands away from your body.

8. Keep the legs strong and the entire torso long, with the abs engaged.

9. Keep your face relaxed and gaze downward as you take at least five breaths.

High-intensity option (figure 7.14)

1. Add more intensity by drawing down through the back of the knees and flexing the feet.

2. As your hips open and flexibility in the lower back develops, you may also choose to grab the ankles or hook the big toes with the first two fingers of each hand.

3. Use each inhale to lengthen the spine and gently pull upward on the toes.

4. Use each exhale to lower your chest more deeply toward the floor.

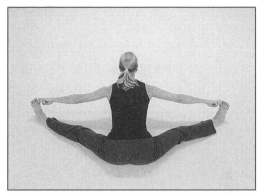

Figure 7.14

Low-intensity option

1. Use a folded blanket under your buttocks to aid in alignment and provide additional comfort.

2. Only walk the hands out as far as you can go comfortably.

Double Pigeon—*opens the hip, relieves sciatica, stretches the spine* (figure 7.15)

1. From Staff pose, bend the left leg in to form a 90-degree angle between the thigh and the shin. Rest that leg on the floor.

2. Bend the right leg and rest it over the left in the same 90-degree angle from the other side. The left shin should be directly under the right one. The left foot should be right under the right knee and the right foot on top of the left knee, forming a triangle with your body as the base.

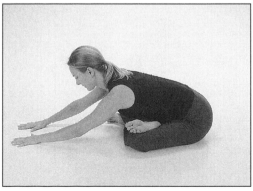

Figure 7.15

3. Use an inhale to realign the spine tall, with sitting bones squarely on the floor.

4. Keep your chest strong, and relax your shoulders down on the exhale.

5. Engage your abs by drawing the navel in and up.

6. Inhale to lengthen while you rest your hands on the floor directly in front of the legs.

7. Exhale as you begin to walk your hands forward, relaxing your body down over the legs. Lower your lengthened torso a little farther down with each exhale.

8. Keep your face relaxed and breath deep.

9. Stay here at least five breaths before moving to the other side.

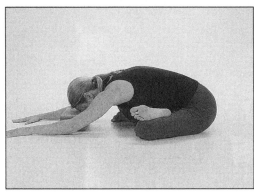

Figure 7.16

High-intensity option (figure 7.16)

1. Make the Triangle posture with your legs and then engage the legs more fully by flexing both feet throughout the pose.

2. As your hip opens, see if you can relax your forehead onto something (a block, your fists, eventually the floor).

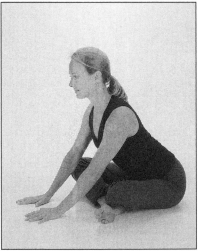

Figure 7.17

Low-intensity option (figure 7.17)

1. Try the posture sitting on your folded blanket.

2. If your legs still won't make the triangle shape without discomfort, simply do the pose with your legs crossed comfortably as you did while you learned the breath.

3. Make sure you still change legs to work both sides.

Kneeling Floor Postures

If you suffer from knee issues, you may choose to eliminate kneeling posture from your practice, or use a folded towel or blanket under your knees.

Camel—*stretches the entire front of the body, particularly the hip flexors; relieves backache; helps improve posture; strengthens the lower back; stimulates the kidneys and thyroid* (Not recommended for students with high blood pressure or lower back problems) (figure 7.18)

1. Come to kneeling with your knees and feet about hip-width apart. Gently press your shins in toward the floor.
2. Make fists with the hands and place them on the lower back at the sacrum.
3. Fully engage the abdominal muscles, scooping your tailbone under and pressing your hips forward.
4. Let your neck stay in line with your spine.
5. Lift your chest upward and allow the back to bend and your head to fall back as you are comfortable.
6. Keep your abs engaged, your buttocks loose, and your face relax as you surrender more into this position.
7. Hold four to five breaths.

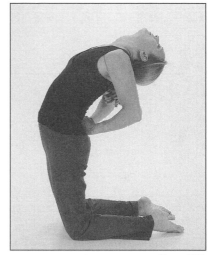

Figure 7.18

High-intensity option
If you feel comfortable in the initial phase of the pose, you may choose one of two other options:
1. Tuck the toes under, with the heels up. Fully engage your abs and scoop the tailbone under. Inhale to lift the chest. Exhale as you slowly and deliberately bend the torso backward and reach for

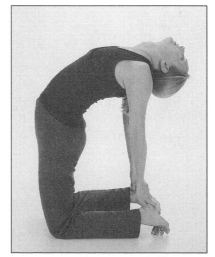

Figure 7.19

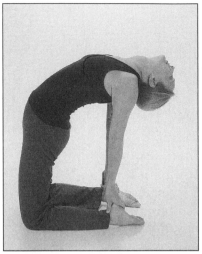

Figure 7.20

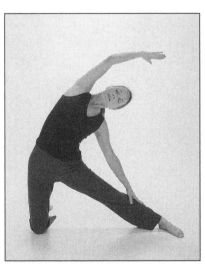

Figure 7.21

the heels with each hand. Be careful with your neck as you try to relax it back (figure 7.19).

2. As your back becomes more flexible, you may choose to leave the front of your foot on the floor and try grasping the heels from this lower position. Be careful not to push yourself beyond where you are ready to go (figure 7.20).

Gate—*stretches the side body, works the obliques, tones the arms and inner thighs, relieves strain in the neck and shoulders* (figure 7.21)

1. Begin in a kneeling position, with your hands resting at your sides, palms facing in.

2. Extend your left foot out to the left side, with the knee and toes turned forward. Let your left toes rest on the floor.

3. Make sure your hips are level and squared to the front of the room. Also notice that the left leg and foot are in line with the left hip.

4. Engage the muscles in the extended leg.

5. On an inhale, raise the right arm to create a long straight line up from right knee to hip to shoulder to fingertips.

6. On the exhale, let the left hand slide down the extended left leg as the right arm arcs overhead toward the left.

7. Keep your hips and shoulders square and your abs fully engaged.

8. Let the right arm continue to arc on each exhale as you extend from the waist. Stop when you feel a nice stretch down the right side of the body.

9. Keep the face relaxed and your gaze steadily forward.

10. Stay here for five breaths before inhaling back up to the center and moving to the other side.

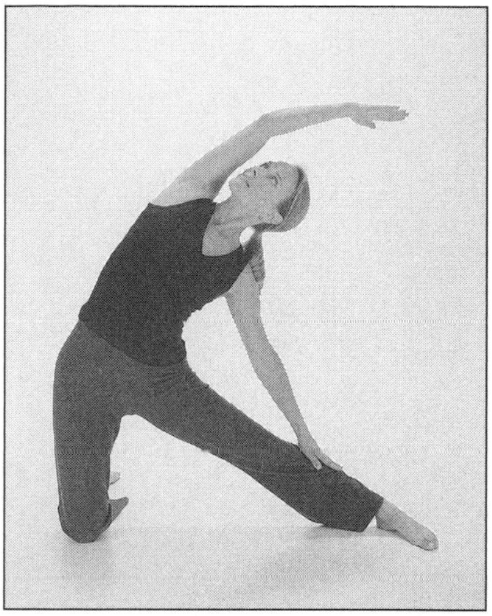

High-intensity option (figure 7.22)
1. On each exhale, look down toward your foot, relaxing the neck.
2. On each inhale, draw the navel farther in and look up toward the extended hand.
3. Let the shoulders square forward a little more with each inhale.

Thread the Needle—*loosens the back, shoulders, and neck; alleviates tightness in the neck and shoulders; refreshes your system* (figure 7.23)

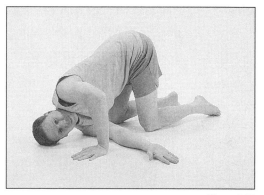

Figure 7.22

1. From kneeling, place the hands on the floor under the shoulders to rest in Tabletop position. Make sure the knees are resting on the floor (or your blanket) directly under the hips.
2. On an inhale, pick up the right hand and raise it out to your side and then up toward the ceiling.
3. On the exhale, lower that arm to thread through the left hand and left knee, reaching the right hand as far through as possible with the palm facing up.

Figure 7.23

4. Rest the right side of the face and the right arm onto the floor while the right shoulder pulls more actively down.
5. Use your left hand for support on the floor.
6. Keep the face relaxed and the abs engaged as you breath deeply here for about five breaths before moving to the other side.

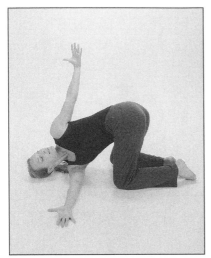

Figure 7.24

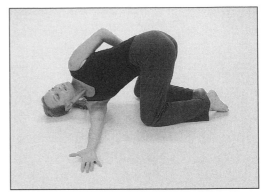

Figure 7.25

High-intensity options (figures 7.24 and 7.25)

1. If you feel like you can rotate farther, instead of using your left arm for support, raise it toward the ceiling and rotate farther onto the back side of the right shoulder and farther to the back of the head rather than the face. If your neck feels OK, then allow your gaze to follow the extended hand (figure 7.24).

2. You may choose to rotate farther by wrapping the extended arm around behind the back and drawing the left shoulder back even more (figure 7.25).

Prone Floor Postures

Postures lying on the belly are not suitable for those who are pregnant. Look for some pose instructions to have modifications more suitable for pregnant students.

Pigeon—*relieves sciatica; opens the hips and chest; stretches the thighs, hip flexors, and hip rotators; stretches muscles around the knee (figure 7.26)*

1. Start from Tabletop position with hands directly under the shoulders and knees under the hips.

2. Pick up the left foot and draw it in toward the chest.

3. With careful movement, lay your left foot in front of your right knee, or for more intensity, open the space behind the knee so that the left foot rests closer to the right hand. The left leg should be at an angle of 90 degrees or less, depending on how this feels to both your hips and your knee.

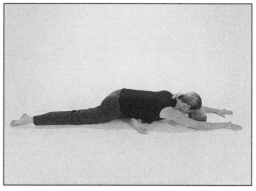

Figure 7.26

4. Slowly slide and lengthen your right leg straight back, resting on the top of the right foot. Place a folded blanket under the right knee if the knee is uncomfortable resting on the floor.

5. On an inhale, walk the hands back to rest under the shoulders as you align the hips and chest to be squared to the front of the room.

6. Open your chest as you raise up tall, resting your shoulders down and relaxing your facial muscles.

7. On an exhale, begin to lower your upper body down toward the floor, leading with the chest.

8. As you draw your upper hip toward the floor, see if you can rest your elbows on the floor or on your block to begin the upper body relaxing.

9. As the upper body relaxes, bring your breath to your hip and continue relaxing both hips into the floor.

10. If you can rest comfortably on your elbows, continue extending the arms outward in front of you. Try resting your forehead on the block. Don't extend farther out or down than you are ready.

11. Keep your breath deep, your face soft, and your gaze downward for at least five deep breaths before coming back to Tabletop to work the other side.

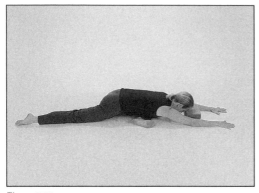

Figure 7.27

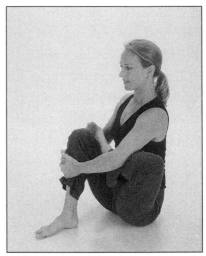

Figure 7.28

High-intensity option (figure 7.27)
While in the Pigeon pose, flex the foot of the bent leg to create greater intensity.

Low-intensity option (figure 7.28)
If Pigeon is uncomfortable for you with the knee at any angle, or if you should not lie on the belly, consider this helpful modification.

1. Rather than starting in Tabletop, have a seat with your legs extended in front of you.

2. Cross the left leg onto the right thigh at the angle that feels right to you.

3. Slowly begin to draw the right leg up toward the chest by bending the knee.

4. Support the right leg with your hands as it comes toward the chest so that the back stays tall. If you have trouble balancing there, rest your hands on the floor behind you, and let the leg come in as it's ready.

5. Keep your gaze forward, your neck and face relaxed, your shoulders down, and your spine long.

Half-Bow—*less intense option to full bow; opens the chest; releases shoulders, hips, and thighs; stimulates the thyroid; strengthens the back and upper arms; works the abs* (figure 7.29)

1. Lie on your belly with your legs extended below you.

2. Rest your chin on the floor and bring both hands to rest under your shoulders, with elbows bent.

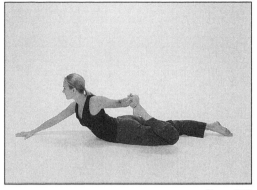

Figure 7.29

3. Bend the left knee and then reach back with the left hand and grab the foot. Start by grabbing the outside of the foot to see how your quadricep and shoulder feel here.

4. If you are comfortable here, slowly push down through the right hand to lift the chest while you also lift the left knee gently.

5. Let the neck stay in alignment with the spine, so your gaze comes up only as you are able to lift the chest.

6. Let your left leg and foot lift as high as you feel comfortable, all the while pressing the foot into the palm of the hand that is holding it.

7. Try to keep the bent leg from straying outward by keeping your thighs parallel, both hips pointed down toward the floor.

8. Keep your face relaxed, your neck and spine long, and your breath deep.

9. Hold for four to five breaths before releasing and moving to the other side.

Low-intensity option (figure 7.30)

1. You may choose to leave your bent knee on the floor to concentrate on lengthening the quadricep before moving on to the rest of the pose.

2. In this case, keep the elbow on the floor rather than pushing up.

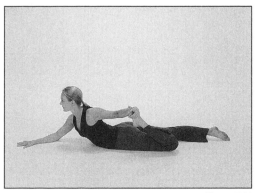

Figure 7.30

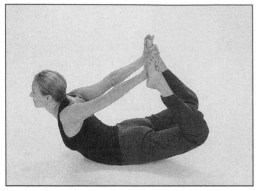

Figure 7.31

Bow—*tones and strengthens the back of the body, stretches and opens the front of the body, works the abs, stimulates digestive process and thyroid activity (This posture is not suitable for those with high blood pressure.)* (figure 7.31)

1. Start by lying on your belly with your legs about hip-width apart and chin resting on the floor.

2. Bend both knees, letting your heels fall back toward your buttocks.

3. On an inhale, reach back with your hands to grasp the outside of the corresponding foot (right hand, right foot). It may be easier to grab one foot at a time or to use a strap wrapped around the front of both feet.

4. On an exhale, engage the abs and press the pubic bone down toward the floor.

5. On an inhale, lift through your upper and lower body, pressing back through your legs to help lift your thighs off the floor.

6. Let the front of your feet push actively into the palm of your hands.

7. Keep your thighs parallel, so that feet are still about hip-width apart.

8. Lift your chest as you feel your shoulder blades drawing together.

9. Use your breath to lift from both ends, keeping your hips and chest level and square.

10. Be sure not to strain the neck, but instead keep it in alignment with the spine and keep the face soft.

11. Stay here four to five breaths before you relax the body down.

Low-intensity option (figure 7.29)
Use Half-Bow as an alternative posture.

Frog—*increases range of motion in the hip joints, releases the muscle and tissue deep within the hips and groin, stretches the upper thigh, improves concentration* (figure 7.32)

1. Turn sideways on your mat, rolling up the ends of the mat to act as extra support under each knee.

2. Come up to Tabletop position, with hands under the shoulders.

3. This time separate the knees to be greater than hip-width apart, resting each

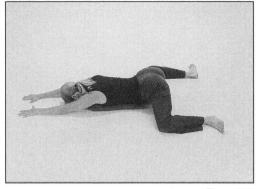

Figure 7.32

on the folded end of the mat. Try to open the legs enough to feel an intense stretch in the hips.

4. See if you can turn the heels out so that the arch of your foot is against the mat. Flex your feet. If you don't feel comfortable turning the feet outward, simply let the top of the foot rest on the floor. Try to create a right angle between the thighs and shins, heels lined up with the knees. I know this is an intense stretch, but it is safe and the rewards are great! Move at your own pace.

5. Slowly begin to see if you can rest down onto your forearms or onto a block, all the while drawing your buttocks back toward the wall behind you.

6. Keep your lower back parallel to the floor by lengthening it and engaging the abs.

7. Scoop your tailbone under.

8. Use each breath to draw down and back.

9. Let your head stay in alignment with your spine and keep your facial muscles soft.

10. After you are here for a little while, attempt to forget the stretch and instead relax into it. Stay here longer than usual to get the relaxation benefit. Using a folded blanket under your chest and belly is another way to help you relax into this intense posture.

11. Breathe here for ten or more breaths before coming up slowly, being careful to lift each knee, rather than slide them.

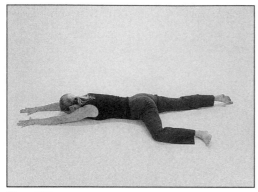
Figure 7.33

Low-intensity option (figure 7.33)

If your hips are extremely tight, you may have difficulty attempting Frog pose. Try this less-intense Half-Frog instead as you work toward full Frog.

1. Lie on your belly with your hands under your shoulders, elbows bent.

2. Use your palm on the floor as support as you lift the left leg out from under you and rest it to your side at a right angle to your body.

3. Create another right angle from your thigh to your shin.

4. Let the foot turn outward, with the arch of the foot resting on the mat.

5. Adjust both hips to face downward onto the floor.

6. Lengthen the right leg below you, and extend the arms to reach out overhead with the palms on the floor.

7. As you breathe, use each exhale to realign your hips, drawing the left more and more toward the floor.

8. Stay here five to ten breaths before returning to the prone position and moving to the other leg.

Supine Floor Postures

Bridge—*encourages flexibility in the back, relieves tension in the neck and shoulders, strengthens the legs and gluts, opens the chest, stretches the ab wall* (figure 7.34)

1. Lie on your back with your knees bent, feet on the floor. Be sure to place the heels directly under the knees to form a 90-degree angle. Make sure the feet and knees are parallel and rest about hip-width apart. To make sure your legs are in the right position, reach down toward your heels with your hands. You should be able to lightly brush the back of your heel with your fingertips.

2. Let your arms rest at your sides, with the palms facing down.

3. Take an inhale to energize the entire body.

4. On the exhale, contract your abs and tilt your pelvis toward the ceiling. Let both feet press evenly onto the floor.

5. On the next inhale, lift your hips and back off the floor until your upper body weight rests in the shoulders. Notice that the weight distributes evenly between the feet and the shoulders by continuing the pressing of the feet onto the floor and also pressing through the upper arms. Keep

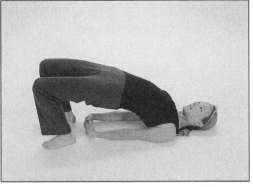

Figure 7.34

your whole foot on the floor, with your big toes carrying as much weight as the little ones.

6. Keep the belly drawing in and the knees parallel.

7. If you feel like you can go a little farther, simply bring the hands together behind the back, linking the fingers. Don't press up onto the back, but instead create more movement upward by tucking each shoulder under the back and lifting the chest. Let the shoulder blades pull in toward one another. Try to create a long line from the shoulders to the knees, to form the "bridge."

8. Expand the ribcage on each inhale, and use the exhale to lift the hips by grounding down farther through the upper arms and feet.

9. Stay here for ten breaths before releasing slowly to the floor, one vertebra at a time. (A slight deviation is helpful for those who suffer from allergies or sinus congestion: to open up the nasal passages, rest the arms on the floor over your head, with palms up, rather than linking fingers behind the back.)

Supine Straddle—*opens the hips, tones the legs, massages the abs* (figure 7.35)

1. Lie flat on your back, bending the knees and drawing them in toward the chest.

2. On an inhale, straighten the legs upward toward the ceiling, leaving your arms resting at your sides.

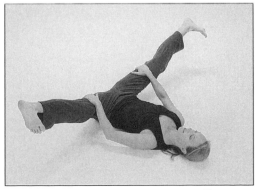

Figure 7.35

3. On an exhale, relax the back into the floor by engaging the abs and releasing each vertebra toward the floor. Inhale and energize the body.

4. On the exhale, open the legs and let them fall outward comfortably while keeping your back, shoulders, and head resting on the floor. Let your legs continue to straddle open farther as you relax the hips on each exhale.

5. Try pressing outward through the balls of the feet for more energy through the legs.

6. You can also rest the hands on the inside of the thighs to encourage more movement (without pushing!). Relax into the openness with each breath.

7. Keep your face, neck, and back relaxed as you take five to ten breaths here.

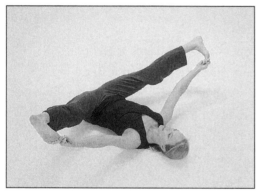

Figure 7.36

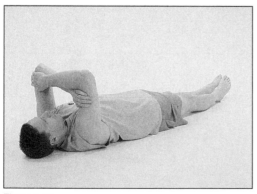

Figure 7.37a

High-intensity option (figure 7.36)

1. As you recline on your back with the legs straddling, see if you can reach out the hands to connect to the big toe on each foot.

2. Hook the first two fingers around the toe as you create energy in the arms and more movement in the legs and hips.

Lying Shoulder Reach—*stretches the shoulders, upper back, and arms (figures 7.37a and 7.37b)*

1. Lie on your back with your legs extended, heels resting on the mat below you. Let your back, shoulders, and head rest on the floor.

2. On an inhale, bring the arms up to form a rectangle by grasping right above the elbow with the opposite hand. Keep the thumbs close to the rest of the fingers rather than wrapping them around the upper arms (figure 7.37a).

3. On an exhale, lead from the right elbow

and draw the rectangle into a diamond shape by dropping the connected arms toward the right side.

4. Pull across as far as your shoulder will reach without letting the upper back come off the floor (figure 7.37b).

5. Inhale back up to center.

6. Use another exhale to drop the connected arms to the left. Continue to move up on each inhale and across on each exhale, letting the shoulder loosen and reach farther with each breath.

7. Keep the face and neck completely relaxed as you stay here for five to ten breaths.

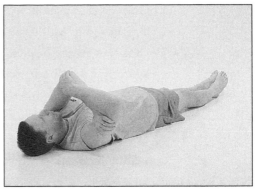

Figure 7.37b

Low-intensity option (figure 7.38)

If it is uncomfortable for you to lie flat and do this position, simply soften the knees with the feet on the floor. This will relieve any pressure you may feel in the back and allow further softening of the back into the floor.

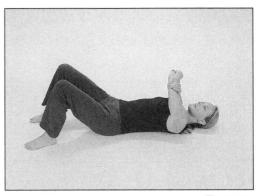

Figure 7.38

Supine Reach Through—*opens the hip, lubricates the hip joints, works the ab, stretches the neck and shoulders* (figure 7.39)

1. As you lie on your back, bend the knees with both feet resting on the floor. Release the back of your head firmly onto the floor.

2. Cross the left leg onto the right thigh, with the outside of the ankle resting just above the right knee. Inhale and energize through to the top of the head.

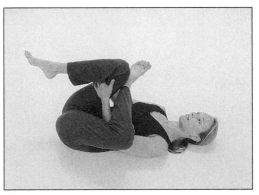

Figure 7.39

3. On the exhale, push off with the right foot and draw the right thigh toward the chest, bringing with it the crossed leg.

4. Without raising the head off the floor, try to reach through the legs to grasp the right thigh with both hands. If your shoulders come off the floor, relax them back down before moving on.

5. Energize on each inhale.

6. Draw the right thigh closer toward the chest on each exhale until you are eventually able to clasp the hands together on the back of the right thigh.

7. Flex both feet.

8. See if you can draw that leg a little farther in with each breath.

9. Keep your face relaxed as you remain here about five breaths before moving to the other leg.

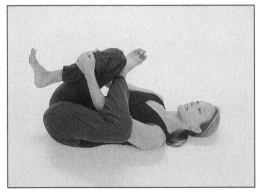

Figure 7.40

High-intensity options (figure 7.40)

1. To add more stretch, try using your left elbow to move your left knee farther open while drawing the right thigh inward.

2. Another option for greater movement is to bend the right knee more so that you can reach past the thigh to the right shin and draw inward from the shin.

Revolving Legs—*stretches and twists the spine, loosens the hips, works the abs, strengthens the legs, builds core strength* (figure 7.41)

1. Lie on your back with your legs extended up toward the ceiling. Keep the feet together and legs strong.

2. Outstretch your arms to either side of you, forming a T with palms down.

3. Relax your head, neck, shoulders, and back onto the floor.

4. Firm the belly, drawing the navel toward the spine.

5. On an inhale, lengthen the legs up through the ball of the foot.

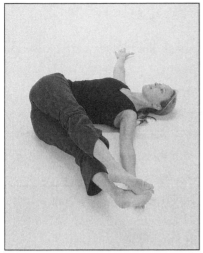

Figure 7.41

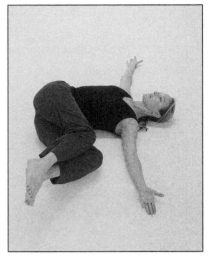

Figure 7.42

6. On an exhale, keep the legs together and let them drop slowly and deliberately toward the left. Let them come just short of touching the floor on the left.

7. Use an inhale to draw the legs slowly back up to center, all the while keeping the belly engaged.

8. Move with the next exhale to lower your legs to the right side, coming just short of resting the legs on the floor.

9. Raise the legs back to center on your next inhale.

10. Continue to let the legs drop side to side with each breath until you have revolved through at least five cycles on each side.

Low-intensity option (figure 7.42)

If keeping the legs straight puts too much strain on your back, do this posture with knees bent. As you cycle down to the side, let the bent knees come close to touching the floor.

Abdominal Isolation Postures

Postures that isolate and tone the abdominals are usually not suitable for those who are pregnant.

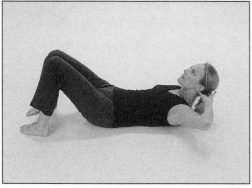

Figure 7.43

Star Gazer—*develops core strength, strengthens back, tones legs and inner thighs* (figure 7.43)

1. Lie on your back, and rest your head and shoulders on the mat.

2. Bend both knees so that your feet are resting comfortably on the floor about hip-width apart.

3. Turn the toes slightly inward, and draw the knees together (a block between the knees is even better).

4. Place your hands behind the head to gently support and cradle the head without pulling on the neck.

5. On an inhale, energize and expand through the chest and back.

6. On an exhale, lift the entire upper body (head, neck, upper back, and mid back if you can get to it) while at the same time contracting the abs and drawing the navel toward the spine.

7. Stay in this lifting position without pulling on the neck as you breathe. You may be able to lift a little more with each exhale, but just don't release lower. Use your ab strength to keep you lifted.

8. Let your gaze be upward as if gazing at the stars. Let your chin stay lifted, your face relaxed, and your knees drawing together and elbows wide.

9. Try to maintain this posture for five to ten breaths.

Descending Legs—*develops core strength, strengthens back, tones legs and arms* (figure 7.44)

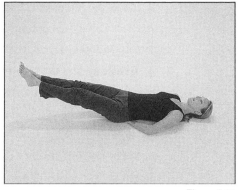

Figure 7.44

1. Lie on your back with legs extended below you.

2. Rest your hands under the lower back with palms facing into the mat.

3. On an inhale, raise both legs together to face toward the ceiling. Make sure your buttocks and lower back are resting into the back of your hands.

4. Keep your head, neck, and shoulders on the floor.

5. Flex your feet, and on a long, slow exhale begin to lower your legs toward the floor, keeping the abs contracted. (Only go as low as you feel you have control of your abs. If you lose control of your abs, your back will arch and be more prone to injury.).

6. Point the toes, and on a long, slow inhale lift the legs back up toward the ceiling.

7. Keep the face relaxed and head resting on the floor.

8. Continue to flow downward on the exhale and upward on the inhale for five to ten breaths. Keep the face relaxed and head resting on the floor.

Low-intensity option

If you are having difficulty maintaining control of your abs, simply keep the legs bent throughout this posture.

Curl with Butterfly Legs—*develops core strength, opens hips, strengthens back, tones arms* (figure 7.45)

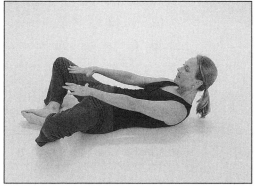

Figure 7.45

1. Lie on your back with legs extended.

2. Bend the knees, and then drop the knees open so that the soles of the feet are together. Keep the feet as close to the groin as possible.

3. Relax the knees open on an exhale or two.

4. Place the hands behind the head to support and cradle it.

5. Inhale and energize the chest and back.

6. Exhale and lift the upper body (head, neck, and as much of the back as you can get off the floor) as you contract your abs, drawing the navel in toward the spine.

7. Inhale as you release back toward the floor, without actually resting all the way down.

8. Make the inhales and exhales as long as you can so that the movement is very slow and controlled.

9. If you felt you could do the posture without supporting the head, then reach the arms out through the legs on each exhale as you curl.

10. Keep the face relaxed as you breathe, and curl for at least ten breaths.

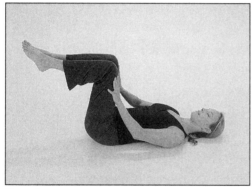

Figure 7.46

Opposing Resistance—*tones abs, develops core strength* (figure 7.46)

1. Lie on the back, resting the head and shoulders on the mat.

2. Bend the knees and bring them in toward the chest until the knees are over the hips.

3. Keeping your head and shoulders on the floor, place your hands onto your thighs.

4. On an inhale, energize through the body.

5. On an exhale, squeeze the navel in toward the spine to engage the abs. As you do, feel the body crunch up slightly.

6. Instead of fully crunching the body, push outward on the thighs with the hands. Create opposite resistance by not letting the legs push away, but instead letting the knees remain over the hips.

7. With the abs contracting, create opposing resistance—pushing out on the thighs, drawing in with the legs.

8. Use your breath to maintain this resistance while relaxing your face and neck.

9. Stay here for at least ten breaths.

Inversions

Inversions vary in difficulty and intensity. Listen to your body to determine if these positions are right for you. Those suffering from eye issues, such as glaucoma or detached retina, should avoid inversions. *Do not perform inversions if you suffer from high blood pressure or heart problems. Women who are pregnant or in the beginning of their menstrual cycles should also avoid some inversions.*

Legs Up the Wall—*relieves swollen and tired feet, develops core strength, improves circulation to legs and hips, calms the nervous system* (figure 7.47)

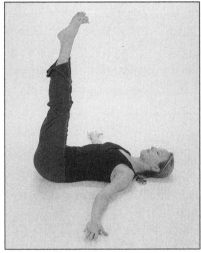

Figure 7.47

This is a safe inversion for everyone!

1. This position may be performed with your legs against the wall or freestanding. (If you use the wall, position your buttocks as close to the wall as you can; then swing your legs up to rest against the wall. Your body would be perpendicular to the wall, with only the soles of the feet and the buttocks touching it.)

2. If you are not actually using a wall for the posture, simply lie on your back with your legs perpendicular to the body and stretched up toward the ceiling.

3. Let your head, shoulders, and back rest comfortably on the floor.

4. Extend arms out from the body in a low V, palms up. Let the back of the hand and the arm rest comfortably on the floor.

5. Draw your navel in toward your spine to engage your abs.

6. Using core strength from your abs and the power of your breath, try to keep the legs extended up, pushing up and out through the balls of both feet.

7. Stay in this pose two to three minutes, breathing deeply.

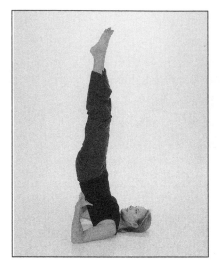

Figure 7.48

Shoulder Stand—*energizes the entire body, helps to work against the negative effects of gravity on the body, refreshes your complexion, improves concentration, increases circulation of blood flow to the brain, stimulates thyroid gland* (figure 7.48)

1. Lie on the back with legs extended below you and your hands at your sides.

2. Keep your head resting on your mat, with your neck long.

3. Press your hands into the floor, and bend your knees in toward the chest on the exhale.

4. On your inhale, roll your hips and buttocks up off the floor. Try to get your hips as high over your shoulders as possible.

5. Place your hands high on your back to support your body.

6. Bend your elbows and rest them on the floor.

7. Squeeze your shoulder blades together to encourage support into the back.

8. As you feel ready, slowly uncurl your legs to reach up vertically.

9. Try to bring the hands even higher on the back and move elbows closer together.

10. With the legs straight up, pull up through the balls of the feet.

11. Do not turn your head, but instead look directly up toward your feet while in this position.

12. For the pose to work effectively, pull your body up as vertical as possible. Weight should be resting in the top of your shoulders, not in your neck.

13. Draw your hips forward and rest as little weight as possible in your hands.

14. Engage your abs.

15. Keep your breath deep and your face relaxed.

16. Stay here for one to three minutes, depending on your level of comfort. If your breathing becomes constricted or too much weight rests in the neck, simply roll down out of the posture at any time. When you are ready to come out, bend the knees and roll down slowly.

Low-intensity options (figure 7.49)

1.If you have any of the conditions listed in the introduction to this section, or just don't feel like going up into full Shoulder Stand, try legs up the wall as your modification.

2. If you want to try Shoulder Stand but your neck doesn't feel comfortable, use your folded blanket to keep the neck from feeling compressed. Place the folded blanket under your neck, shoulders, and mid-back so that the top of your shoulders rests about three inches from the top edge of the blanket. When you roll up, the shoulders will be positioned on the edge of the blanket.

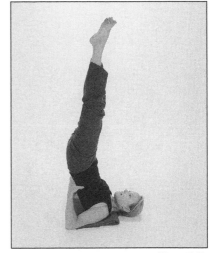

Figure 7.49

Candlestick—*the same as the shoulder stand; however, the posture also stretches the back and hamstrings* (figure 7.50)

1. Follow same instructions as performing Shoulder Stand.

2. After getting into Shoulder Stand, firm the belly and bend the knees down toward the forehead. If the knees fall closer to the chin than the forehead, bring your hips farther up.

3. Keep the feet close together, with the toes pointing up toward the ceiling.

4. Continue to support the back with your hands.

5. Keep the neck long and the face relaxed.

6. Do not move your head in this position, but keep your gaze focused on your toes.

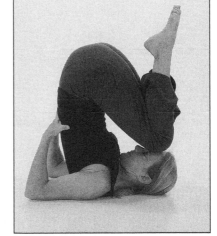

Figure 7.50

7. Stay here one to three minutes, depending on your level of comfort. Release your hands and roll down slowly when you are ready to come out.

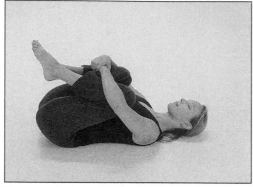

Figure 7.51

Low-intensity option (figure 7.51)

If you choose to forego inversions, try this comforting modification of hugging the knees.

1. From lying on your back, draw your knees into your chest.

2. Wrap the arms around the knees, bringing them closer to the chest.

3. Keep the knees together and moving inward on each exhale.

4. Keep your head and shoulders resting on the floor.

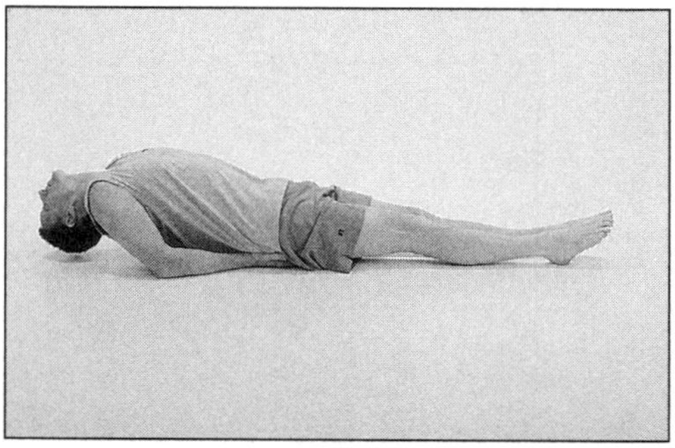

Figure 7.52

Fish—*tones the upper chest, relieves tension in the neck and shoulders, stretches the neck, stimulates the thyroid, stretches the legs and toes, improves lung capacity* (figure 7.52)

Fish pose is a wonderful counterpose to both Shoulder Stand and Candlestick.

1. Start by lying on the floor with hands tucked under the buttocks, palms down.

2. Bring your elbows as close together as possible underneath you.

3. Keep your feet together and your knees straight and parallel to one another.

4. Inhale and lift onto your elbows.

5. Tuck your head under so that the crown of your head rests gently on the floor. Your elbows should be tucked in enough that they take the weight, rather than your neck and head.

6. Open your throat by tilting the chin back and looking behind you.

7. Lift up on each inhale from your heart center. Visualize that your breastbone is being drawn toward the ceiling.

8. Keep your facial muscles and neck completely relaxed, and breathe here for five to ten breaths.

9. Be very deliberate as you come out of the posture by first lifting up onto your elbows, bringing the head up slowly and then returning your back to the floor.

Low-intensity option (figure 7.53)
If you suffer from neck problems, try the pose with the neck lifted from the floor, rather than dropping back. Continue to lift from the chest, but keep the neck long and lifted.

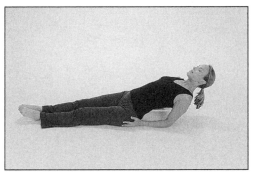

Figure 7.53

Prayer for Removing Barriers

"Search me, O God, and know my heart; test me and know my thoughts. Point out anything in me that offends you, and lead me along the path of everlasting life" (Psalm 139:23–24).

Part 3

Stillness

chapter 8

Achieving Rest

REST IS SO MUCH MORE THAN INACTIVITY. IN FACT, *RANDOM HOUSE DICTIONARY* LISTS thirty-seven definitions for the word *rest*. Some of them are "relief or freedom, especially from troubles or exertion," "a mental or spiritual calm; tranquility," and "to be quiet or still."

As we've discussed, you cannot avoid struggle. In fact, God says you should welcome it as an opportunity for growth and development in your faith. So how do you achieve a mental and spiritual calm in the face of hardship, loss, and pain? You can't always walk away. You can't seem to forget. And you certainly can't get over the fact that life is just not fair.

You achieve rest not just by working through your problems to a tidy resolution, but by relinquishing control of those issues to God. Notice again what Paul says in Philippians 4:6–7, but this time pay careful attention to what He promises. "Don't worry about anything; instead, pray about everything. Tell God what you need, and thank him for all he has done. If you do this, you will experience God's peace, which is far more wonderful than the human mind can understand. His peace will guard your hearts and minds as you live in Christ Jesus."

True rest, true peace, does not come from problem resolution or from positive thinking. God's peace, the only true and lasting peace, comes from knowing that God is in control and allowing that control to have lordship in your life.

Throw Out the Agenda

If you've ever attended a town council meeting or a city planning meeting, you know that the agenda is everything. It rules from the minute the group assembles to its dismissal. Usually, nothing is discussed that isn't represented in some way on the agenda.

But what if someone unexpectedly attended the meeting, someone who had big ideas and great plans that this town had never considered? What if this guest could offer a long-range plan that would change the course of this town's future, taking it far beyond the dream of any of the council members?

What a tragic loss it would be if our response was, "Sorry, you're not on the agenda. There's no time for your proposal. There's no space in our busy schedule. I already have it all planned out, and you're not a part of my vision." If you are ever to experience God's peace, you must first accept that God's plan for you is far greater than anything you could hope to accomplish alone. Therefore, the first step to accepting the peace He offers is to lay aside your own desires, your personal agenda, the expectations you have for yourself and for others. Let go of judgments you have made about your own abilities and judgments you have made about others. Try to see yourself and those around you as blank pages with open agendas.

How is God to use you if your pages are full and written in indelible ink? Try leaving the story of your life open for rewrites, mark-throughs, and erasures. Leave some of the pages blank altogether so that God can create for you a story of fruitfulness, love, and service. Begin to visualize your life, not as you've planned it, but as God sees it—with limitless possibilities.

In leaving yourself open and available to God's plan, you are demonstrating your trust and faithfulness in Him. You are also freeing yourself of the worries and anxieties that accompany those full pages. You are creating a restful heart, one that has found relief from the struggles and troubles of life.

Lay Down Your Baggage

The second step in experiencing the full peace of God is to lay down all the emotional baggage of your past. Not only should your future be God's, but also your past.

Don't think you're carrying any extra baggage? Check your bags against the ones mentioned by Max Lucado in his book *Traveling Light*: "The suitcase of guilt. A sack of discontent. You drape a duffel bag of weariness on one shoulder and a hanging bag of grief on the other. Add on a backpack of doubt, an overnight bag of loneliness, and a trunk of fear. Pretty soon you're pulling more stuff than a skycap. No wonder you're so tired at the end of the day. Lugging baggage is exhausting."[1]

The emotional baggage of your past is exhausting to both your heart and body. Physically, carrying old baggage can cause you to experience an unhealthy appetite, lethargy, depression, anxiety, and much more. Spiritually, unchecked baggage from your past can create a bitterness toward God, a lack of joy, and a hardened heart.

God doesn't ask us to carry this load, but instead instructs us to drop those suitcases at His feet. "Come to me," He invites, "all of you who are weary and carry heavy burdens, and I will give you rest" (Matthew 11:28). For Him, the load is easy; for us, it can seem an insurmountable weight because these are bags we are not meant to carry. Finding relief and rest from the past that haunts you comes simply from letting it go. Take inventory of your past. Learn from your mistakes. Be thankful that those experiences have made you

_____ (stronger, more attentive, more resilient, more faithful—you fill in the blank). Then move on. Let it go. Learn to rest in the quiet of a past that is truly history.

In *Living Prayer*, Robert Benson suggests that the longer we hold on to the old, "the longer it holds on to us, and the longer it keeps us from hearing the Word that we so long to hear. It becomes a matter of not being able to hear God's voice because we are so full of our own. We cannot be filled with God until we are not so full of ourselves. Our hearts and minds, wonderful as they are, are simply too small. We cannot give our hearts to God, or anyone else for that matter, as long as they are too heavy for us to lift."[2]

Look to Someone Bigger

You will never find rest if you choose to focus on the struggles of your own life. In doing so, those troubles get bigger and bigger, becoming magnified in your own self-importance. Achieving rest comes from letting go of your personal agenda, setting down your past hurts, and then looking toward God to find your worth and purpose.

In God's magnificence we become small. In accepting His gifts of love, peace, and joy, we become awed. In the presence of God's power, we become humbled. Peter writes in 1 Peter 5:6–7, "So humble yourselves under the mighty power of God, and in his good time he will honor you. Give all your worries and cares to God, for he cares about what happens to you."

Now that's rest. We find comfort and assurance in the fact that God cares about us. Why do we have to worry about anything when we have the Creator of the universe watching our backs?

When you let go of your own issues long enough to really consider God, His power, His love, and the works of His hands, then you can no longer look at yourself the same way. He is so big, and we are so small, yet still so important to Him, it's truly mind-boggling.

So rest comes from the freedom to be who God made you. You can stop trying to be what you're not, stop trying to live up to some worldly standard of what you expect yourself to be, stop thinking of yourself as the sum total of your past. Instead you can look to Someone so much bigger than yourself and find your worth and purpose in light of His plan.

Readying Your Body for Rest

Just as you ready your heart for life in Christ through letting go, you ready your body for rest in much the same way. Start by relinquishing any expectations you had for practicing yoga and whether you "meet them" or not. Instead, notice how you feel right now and be thankful for any progress that you will make. Progress may be found with your body's conditioning, your breath's development, or your overall perspective and attitude. Your greatest progress may come simply from allowing yourself to get quiet for whatever length of time you practice.

Readying yourself for rest is a very important transition from poses to relaxation and meditation. Your purpose here is to make the necessary adjustments to your body and environment to allow yourself to lie comfortably on the floor during relaxation. Therefore, it is vital that you take physical inventory of how you are feeling after you complete your final posture.

If, for example, you've chosen a flow of postures that works vigorously on the back, you may find your back to be sensitive and uncomfortable lying flat on the mat. Likewise, if you practiced in a room that was a comfortable temperature to you as you practiced your heat-building postures, then it is probably going to be too cool for you as you relax. These are the type of things, both physically and environmentally, that you want to assess as you prepare to relax. The purpose of relaxation is to prepare your heart for meditation and to allow your body to absorb all the benefits of the previous poses. Think of your relaxation posture as the Save key on the computer of your body. The information can be typed in, but if you don't finish with the Save key, the information can't be retrieved and is of little, if any, use.

Ironically, for new yoga students, it seems that relaxation is the hardest part to master because we have structured our lives to be on the go all the time. Over and over, I watch new students packing up to leave as we begin relaxation.

Don't fall into the trap of thinking you have to be moving for exercise to be beneficial. Let your relaxation period benefit you physically as you assimilate the changes your body has experienced. Let it benefit you emotionally as you settle into possibly the only few minutes of peace and quiet you will get in a day. And let it benefit you spiritually as you retrain your heart to be still and listen for God's voice.

Start with a minimum of five minutes of relaxation at the end of your practice session. Then as your practice develops, add more time to relax and meditate.

Finishing Postures

As you notice how your body is feeling, there may be a couple of finishing postures you will need to perform to make you more comfortable. It is my recommendation that you perform at least the first two postures described below at the end of every practice. They will help ensure a healthy back and a greater degree of comfort lying on the floor. Choose from the other postures as needed.

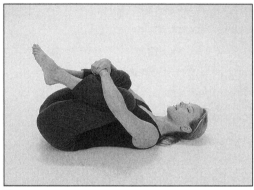
Figure 8.1

Hugging the Knees—*particularly helpful if the lower back is sensitive, stretches the lower back, massages the entire back* (figure 8.1)

1. Lie on your back with legs extended and head resting comfortably on the mat.

2. Bend both knees and bring them in toward the chest. Keep them comfortably close together as you draw them in.

3. Wrap your arms around both shins, connecting the hands around the legs if possible. Gently draw the legs farther inward on the exhale.

4. Stay here, drawing the legs in, or roll slowly and gently from side to side to massage the lower back.

5. Let the head stay on the floor, but follow the direction of the body.

6. Keep the face relaxed as you stay in this posture as long as is necessary to relieve any sensitivity in the back.

Visualization

As you enjoy the comforting benefits of this pose, visualize your body lying in God's open hand. As you curl your legs in, imagine the fingers of God wrapping around you to hold you in His constant and unfailing love. Enjoy the feeling of being surrounded by His love.

Lying Spinal Twist—*relieves tension in the back, neck, and hips* (figure 8.2)

1. Lie on your back with your legs extended, head resting on the floor.

2. On an inhale, bend the right leg and draw it in toward the chest.

3. Place your left hand on the top of your right knee.

4. On an exhale, use the left hand to guide the right knee down toward the floor on the left side. Let it drop as far toward the floor as it will go comfortably, without pulling on it at all.

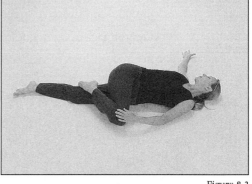

Figure 8.2

5. Reach back toward the right with the right hand, and draw the right shoulder toward the floor.

6. Try to create equal twisting across and down from the leg and back and down from the shoulder.

7. If your neck permits, turn and look out over the right shoulder while keeping the head on the floor and face relaxed.

8. Breathe deeply as you remain here as long as is necessary to feel any residual tension release.

9. When you're ready to move to the other side, bring your leg back up to center on the inhale and then release it back to the floor on the exhale.

Lying Knee Circles—*relieves tension in the spine and buttocks, loosens the hips* (figure 8.3)

1. Lie on your back with the head resting on the floor.

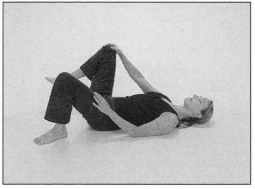

Figure 8.3

2. Bend both knees and bring them in toward the chest.

3. Place one hand on either knee.

4. Separate the knees slightly and make small circles with each knee, one at a time, until the hip joint feels comfortable. Let the movement gently massage the hip and sacrum into the floor.

5. Keep the face and neck relaxed as you stay here until the hips feel loose and comfortable.

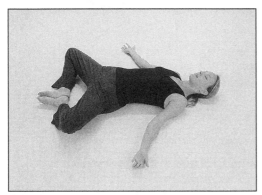

Figure 8.4

Supine Butterfly—*loosens the hips* (figure 8.4)

1. Lie on your back, bringing the soles of the feet together so that the knees drop outward to either side.

2. Keep your head and neck relaxed onto the floor.

3. With each exhale try to relax your hips more open, while you relax your back down into the floor.

4. Breathe into any place that feels tight as you stay here as long as necessary to feel more openness and comfort.

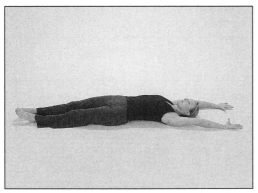

Figure 8.5

Total Body Reach—*loosens the arms, legs, torso, hips, and spine; improves circulation* (figure 8.5)

1. Lie on your back with the entire back side of your body resting on the floor.

2. Use an inhale to bring the arms overhead and lay your hands, palms up, on the mat.

3. Use an exhale to lengthen the body in the opposite direction by pulling out through the spine and down through the toes.

4. Continue to stretch in both directions as

you spread your fingers, point the toes, and engage the face by opening the eyes and jaw wide.

5. Stay here for as many breaths as it takes to engage the body fully before using an exhale to release the arms and relax completely into the mat.

Relaxation Postures

Once the body feels comfortable on the floor, you are ready to get into your relaxation posture. We will talk more about the purpose of staying in relaxation in the following chapter, but for now let's look at the practical application of getting into a restful position.

Environmental Concerns

Notice the following before you lie down for relaxation:

1. Is the room a comfortable temperature? Remember that your body temperature will drop rather dramatically when you lie down to relax. The last thing you want to do is fight the cold room for your focus.

2. If you don't have control over the temperature of the room, do you have an adequate jacket or blanket to use as a cover-up? Think primarily about covering your chest and feet.

3. Is the surface you're lying on comfortable? Double your mat if necessary or lie on a blanket.

4. Have you eliminated as many of the distractions as possible? Try to practice when the kids are napping or the construction crew next door is on break. Close whatever doors you can. Turn off the lights. If you've been practicing with music, turn it off or down very low.

Physical Concerns

Once the room is ready and your body is prepared, get into whichever of these relaxation postures is the most comfortable for you. Each of these postures is designed to help you relax, but also to be your final demonstration of openness and receptivity. Let the palms up, in particular, be a reminder of the letting go in order to give yourself entirely to God's purpose.

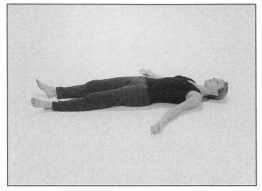

Figure 8.6

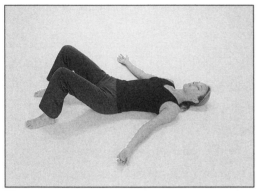

Figure 8.7

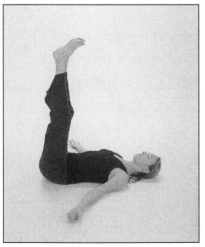

Figure 8.8

Corpse (figure 8.6)

Lie on your back with the legs extended. Let the toes drop out comfortably as you release the legs. Let the arms rest on the floor at a comfortable distance from your sides, palms facing up. Make sure the neck is long and the chin is not higher than your forehead. (Place a small towel under the neck, if that helps.) Close your eyes and breathe deeply. You may also consider placing your folded blanket under the knees for additional help in relaxing.

Knees Raised (figure 8.7)

Lie on your back with the feet on the floor, knees up. Let your feet rest comfortably on the floor to relieve any pressure you may feel in your back. Again, hands are at your sides, palms up. Face is relaxed and breath is deep.

Legs Up the Wall (figure 8.8)

Position your upper body perpendicular to the wall, with the legs resting up the wall. Relax your back onto the floor as the hands are at your sides, palms up. Keep the face relaxed and breathe deeply.

Relaxation Breath

You will experience much of the relaxing benefit of the breath when you master and maintain the complete breath we use in yoga. The complete breath is designed to create a unity of energy (inhale) and relaxation (exhale), so it serves the overall purpose of the practice well.

However, as we move into the resting portion of a session, more emphasis can be placed on the part of the breath that facilitates relaxation—the exhale. As you get into your comfortable position, take note of your breath again. Make sure that you are still breathing through the nose, deeply and freely.

Then slowly begin to transition more length to the exhale in an effort to enhance the restful feeling of the body. Counting the beats of the breath can be distracting, but for the purposes of learning this breath, let's use the count as an illustration.

If you, for example, had a complete breath of six counts in (inhale) and six counts out (exhale), you would begin to modify to six counts in and seven counts out. The next breath would continue with six counts in and eight counts out. Follow this pattern of lengthening the exhale until you are able to have a count on the exhale of double the inhale.

Try to follow the long exhale as the breath moves down the body as if it is leaving out the bottom of the feet, and with it any tension or tightness that might be left in your system. As you continue this pattern of breathing, think about the life brought in on the inhale. Let the exhale seep out slowly as if you want to hang on to the life in that breath as long as possible. Feel all the muscles soften with the long exhale. Feel each vertebrae as they melt one by one toward the floor. Once you have let go completely, you are ready to bring your focus away from the body and toward the thoughts of your heart—also known as meditation.

Prayer for Rest

"I know the Lord is always with me. I will not be shaken, for He is right beside me. No wonder my heart is filled with joy, and my mouth shouts His praises! My body rests in hope. You have shown me the way of life, and you will give me wonderful joy in your presence" (Acts 2:25–26, 28).

chapter 9

Hearing the Whisper

So you've breathed, stretched, bent, and twisted. You've even calmed and quieted. But now you're lying on the floor, and all that comes to mind is . . . the grocery list, the overdue library book, the job, the kids, a hangnail . . . you name it. Everything wants time in your thoughts as you lie quietly. You look at your watch. *What?! It's only been thirty seconds? It feels like thirty minutes!*

Don't give up. God's Word instructs you clearly here. He simply says to "wait." If you ever want to know God's heart, you have to learn to wait. Everything that you've done up to this point in your Christ-centered yoga practice is preparing you for this moment when you wait.

Psalm 37:7 instructs you to "be still in the presence of the LORD, and wait patiently for him to act." Notice that the posture of waiting is still, quiet, and patient. Yet waiting for God is anything but passive. In fact, it is considered an attitude of watchfulness. It carries a sense of expectancy and anticipation. We know that God's time is not our time, yet we know God's promise is to listen and respond. So we wait, knowing that it will bring results.

"I waited patiently for the LORD to help me, and he turned to me and heard my cry" (Psalm 40:1). When you wait, God can work. When you rush, you are telling God that you can rely on your own strength, your own wisdom, and your own power. "But those who wait on the LORD will find new strength. They will fly high on wings like eagles. They will run and not grow weary. They will walk and not faint" (Isaiah 40:31). Remember, you are not waiting on yourself or some opportunity, but on God. It is from His work that you receive strength beyond your own power.

You'll wait thirty minutes for a pizza, three weeks for the new outfit you ordered online, two years for your bangs to grow out. Can you wait with the same anticipation for the Lord to act, to speak, to respond? Your body is ready, and your mind is clear and focused. Use this time of relaxation on your mat as an opportunity to physically, emotionally, and spiritually wait on the Lord.

Waiting cultivates a quiet heart and a teachable spirit. But like any other new skill, don't expect it to happen overnight. Start with a waiting period of quiet and meditation that lasts at least ten minutes. Try to lengthen this portion of class as you develop an attitude of watchful expectancy to last twenty to thirty minutes. Remember that God is not timing you; He simply wants to talk with you.

Waiting to Hear

There are two ways I will encourage you to use this time on your mat: either in silent listening or in quiet meditation.

I believe that listening (and not just to God) is quickly becoming a lost art. As quickly as conversation begins, many of us are thinking ahead to the next witty remark or thought-provoking comment we will make. "Oh, did you say something? I was too busy trying to be interesting to actually hear what you had to say." I know I'm guilty of this. I'll ask, "How are you?" Then I don't even stay around long enough to hear the answer. We do the same thing with God. "Hi, God, checking in because I promised myself I'd do twenty minutes of prayer a day. (Deep breath.) OK, here goes: please help Aunt Mae, cousin Henry, watch over the children, bring peace to the Middle East . . ."

Do you give God any time to get a word in? Someone said to me that God gave us one mouth and two ears; therefore, we should listen twice as much as we talk. Good theory. Have you tried it?

Many of us are just plain uncomfortable with the silence of listening. An uncomfortable silence, a pregnant pause, leaves us feeling like we haven't prepared, haven't examined ourselves enough, aren't grateful enough, or aren't being sympathetic to the needs of others.

Certainly God wants to hear from you, but He also wants to speak to you. Jesus told the religious leaders who asked if He was the Messiah, "My sheep recognize my voice; I know them, and they follow me" (John 10:27). You recognize His voice by spending quality time with Him. You draw near. You abide. And in that closeness, that quiet, He speaks. You can call it "leadings," "promptings," "inner testimony," or "a chat among friends." But listening to God speak to you through the Holy Spirit is essential to leading a Spirit-guided, Christ-centered life.

Claire Cloninger, in her book *The Kaleidoscope,* reminds us that even Jesus, the Son of God, needed regular times of silence in God's presence. "He came to do only what His Father revealed to Him in secret (John 5:19–20, 30). And so hearing that still, small voice was vital to His life and ministry. Luke's Gospel tells us that 'He himself would often slip away to the wilderness and pray' (Luke 5:16). If Jesus needed quiet times of communion with the Father, how much more do we. Only by pulling away into our hidden hearts to listen for the voice of our God can we experience Him deeply. There is a special room prepared within the heart of each believer which can only be unlocked by the key of silence. When we are willing to sit still, expectantly waiting, He will meet us there."[1]

Therefore, the first step to hearing is to be quiet. Matt Redman also talks about the importance of silence in worship in his book *Facedown.* "Moments of stillness take us even deeper into Him, creating essential space for us to hear the voice of God. As we quiet our souls in response to His glory, they are opened further to perceive even more of His holy radiance. In stillness we both honour and behold God. The God of glory, who thunders over the mighty waters, reveals Himself intimately and quietly to the depths of our hearts. When alone, and when gathered as a worship community, we must learn to listen out for Him—in the sound of sheer silence."[2]

How Are You Listening?

Just as you worship with your whole body, you must listen with your whole heart. Too often we sit (or lie) down with the best of intentions, but our minds immediately begin to wander. To hear God speak, you must be completely present in the moment. You have set aside the baggage of your past and thrown out the agenda of your future; now you are ready to bask in the comforting glow of the presence of God.

Transform the way you listen:

1. Are you listening with expectation? You can anticipate His speaking to you based on His unmatched reliability.
2. Are you listening with a quiet spirit? It's time to let Him do some of the talking.
3. Are you listening patiently? As you wait, possibly God is changing and preparing you for His message and His answer.
4. Are you listening confidently? Know that God will answer.
5. Are you listening dependently? Come to Him recognizing that you are totally dependent on the Holy Spirit for revealing truth.
6. Are you listening submissively? You must accept that God's answer is not always the one you hope for or expect.
7. Are you listening attentively? Let God have your full focus.
8. Are you listening carefully? Learn to discern God's truth from error.
9. Are you listening gratefully? Come to Him with a thankful heart.
10. Are you listening reverently? We should be humbled that this same omnipotent God is willing to listen to us, while simultaneously giving direction to the universe.

To improve the quality of your listening, I suggest that you consider one of these ten listening characteristics each time you come to the mat for prayer and meditation. For example, on the first session, fully consider if you are coming before God with expectation that He will respond. Do you really believe that the Holy Spirit speaks for God? Do you honestly believe that you can hear God's voice in some audible or inaudible way? Do you think God only spoke to those alive during biblical times? Be honest with yourself.

Continue a personal examination of each of these characteristics when you get to the mat at the end of each session. As you dissect how you listen, you may uncover some barriers that have impeded you from actually hearing God speak. You may uncover some questions that you will need to check against Scripture or consult with your clergy. But don't let the process go unexamined—cultivate a quiet heart that listens in the silence.

God has a purpose for your life. God has a plan for your success in His kingdom. He has guidance for your present situation. He is waiting to tell you, waiting for the opportunity to share with you this incredible news. But He's been known to speak in a whisper. And He's not willing to talk over the noise of your life. What will you sacrifice to hear Him?

Quiet Meditation

As you lie still and quiet on your mat, the other opportunity you have besides listening in silence is meditation. For many, the word *meditation* may have a mystical connotation. You may visualize someone sitting cross-legged with hands resting on their knees chanting, "Ohm." For some, this is meditation.

But for a Christ-centered practice, meditation is once again an opportunity to honor God. The word itself simply means "reflection" or "contemplation." It is found in the Bible numerous times—more than fifty in the Old Testament alone. Here are a few examples:

o "Study the Book of the Law continually. Meditate on it day and night so that you may be sure to obey all that is written in it" (Joshua 1:8).

o "The one thing I ask of the LORD—the one thing I seek most—is to live in the house of the LORD all the days of my life, delighting in the LORD's perfections and meditating in his temple" (Psalm 27:4).

o "I lie awake thinking of you, meditating on you through the night" (Psalm 63:6).

○ "I will meditate on your principles" (Psalm 119:23)

○ "O God, we meditate on your unfailing love as we worship in your Temple" (Psalm 48:9).

God wants your focus and your thoughts; therefore, He is glorified when you meditate on Him. Meditation is a single-mindedness of thought toward one thing. So meditating on God may one day mean reflecting on His forgiveness, the price that was paid, the sacrifice, our unworthiness. On another day, it may mean single-mindedness of thought regarding God's love—its unfailing, unchanging, unconditional nature, and so on.

With your body quiet and your mind focused from the yoga practice, you will have a clarity to share with God your uncluttered thoughts, free from distraction and influence from others. You may be able to see more clearly your blessings, enabling you to praise Him with a thankful heart. You may even see more clearly how God may be using your struggle, resulting in growth and ultimately joy. The practice may also provide you a new level of concentration that will prolong your intimacy with God, allowing you to experience a deeper level of closeness and relationship.

In essence, you are giving God quality time—not leftover time, and not time on the run. You are giving God your best, coming to Him with a still posture, a clear mind, and a prepared heart.

In *Meditative Prayer* Richard Foster calls meditation "sinking down into the light and life of Christ and becoming comfortable in that posture." He explains that in practicing meditation, "we create the emotional and spiritual space which allows Christ to construct an inner sanctuary in the heart" (in much the same way we are creating physical space in the practice). He goes on to write that this practice transforms the inner personality because "we cannot burn the eternal flame of the inner sanctuary and remain the same." Second, he believes that "meditation will send us into our ordinary world with greater perspective and balance. As we learn to listen to the Lord, we gain new practical handles on life's ordinary problems."[3]

To effectively bring your focus from the practice to meditation, I would encourage you to determine your meditation direction at the beginning of the session, knowing that God may have another direction for your thoughts. If so, don't fight to use your agenda; go with God's. Pattern that session's practice around your meditation focus, with your postures, attitude, and breath of prayer reflecting the theme. For example, if you are considering meditating on the comfort of God's presence, you may select restorative poses with little strength required and a scriptural prayer, such as "Let your unfailing love surround us, LORD, for our hope is in you alone" (Psalm 33:22).

By doing so, your quiet time of meditation should flow easily from postures to stillness. Even if you choose meditation over silence, remember that God may use your focus to speak to you. Be ready to get quiet and listen.

Start your meditation time from the comfortable relaxation pose you selected. Focus first on your breathing, noticing the pattern of inhalations and exhalations. Begin to lengthen your exhale, possibly to be twice as long as the length of the inhale.

Visualizations

From here, you have several options for guiding your meditation time. If you continue to struggle with distractions, visualizations can be helpful tools to keep your mind God-focused. I would encourage you to keep your eyes closed but focus with your imagination on a symbol of your spirituality.

You may choose to picture an object such as cross or a flame, reflecting on what that image means to your faith. You might visualize a birth (a new beginning) or a death (also a new beginning!) as a way to focus your thoughts.

You may want to visualize a scene in which Jesus is present, such as the Sermon on the Mount or His crucifixion. Taking it to a more personal level, you might visualize a scene in which Jesus is present with you as you lie meditating. Perhaps He takes your hand as you stretch it open. Perhaps you feel Him as the mat, being your foundation to hold you up and protect you from falling. Or perhaps you can visualize Jesus as the comforting blanket that covers you, bringing you a warmth that fills your whole body, your Immanuel. You could meditate on your dependency on Christ by visualizing yourself as the branch and Jesus as the vine. The branch clings to (abides in) the vine with complete dependency—literally clinging to the vine for life. Separated, it wilts and dies. Connected, it is nourished and fruitful. Visualize not only the vine and branch, but the colors and fragrances that accompany a fruitful branch. Feel the fullness and nourishment that comes from Christ.

Find an image that works for you in keeping you focused and Christ-centered. There are endless possibilities, but potentially only one (or none) that works for you. Remember that these images are not the ultimate goal of your meditation. They are simply a method by which you can further direct your attention toward prayer.

Don't be afraid to use your imagination. It is a gift from God that comes hardwired as part of your full package at creation.

Getting "Washed in the Word"

Another method for guiding your meditation time is to meditate on God's Word. This practice will not only allow you to hide God's Word in your heart, but also keep your mind from wandering and losing its single-mindedness.

John Ortberg, in his book *The Life You've Always Wanted,* calls this immersion into Scripture being "washed in the Word." He describes what happens when something gets washed. "Soap and water move through the fibers of the dirty fabric at the deepest level, lifting out the impurities and removing them. Only after the washing can we see the fabric in the state for which it was originally designed. When we come to God, our minds and hearts are like that, cluttered with false beliefs and attitudes, deadly feelings, misguided plans and hopes and fears."

He goes on to write that when our minds are "washed by the Word," then we are transformed by it, our minds are renewed. As God creates a clean heart and a right spirit within us, our minds are filled with thoughts and feelings of truth, love, joy, and humility. In essence, every moment becomes, as Ortberg says, "a miniature reflection of life in the Kingdom of God."[4]

So as you lie ready for meditation, if your thoughts don't automatically flow into ceaseless praise, consider meditating on Scripture as an opportunity to guide the mind and equip the soul.

Here are some helpful tips John Ortberg offers to get you started:

1. Ask God to meet you in Scripture. Ask Him to begin to wash your mind. Be open to the possibility that God is speaking to you through His Word.
2. Read the Scripture with a repentant spirit, ready to surrender anything. Read it with an obedient and vulnerable heart.
3. Meditate on a brief passage. Read it slowly, allowing the words to sink into your heart.
4. Take one thought or verse with you through the day. What the mind repeats, it retains. For one day, live with these words.
5. Allow this thought to become part of your memory. Transform your mind by "hiding God's Word in your heart."[5]

Robert Benson describes a similar process called "sacred reading," or *lectio divina*. "You begin by reading a Scripture passage slowly, aloud perhaps, once or twice or three times. Then you imagine yourself in the setting of the scripture itself. You see yourself as the different characters in the story or the setting, you listen to the sounds that emanate from it, touch its textures, smell its smells, feel its tensions. Then you begin to listen for what it is saying to you. The hearing is prayer itself. The hearing is the beginning of being 'shaped by the Word.'" Here, he says, is where meditation, or *meditatio*, begins, in which the Scripture "starts to work on you rather than you on it."[6]

Just Pray!

Remember that your quiet meditation time is not about the method but about drawing near to God. During this time, you may feel God leading you to simply come to Him in unscripted prayer, sharing your adoration, your concerns, and your repentance. You may have issues that can now come to the surface to be turned over to Christ's lordship and authority.

Talk to God as you would your closest friend—with honesty, enthusiasm, and openness. Don't worry about having the right words to say. God doesn't necessarily need poetry from you. He just wants you to bring yourself to Him, stutters and all, knowing that He is the only one worthy, willing, and able to hear and answer the prayers of your heart.

Think of prayer as an awesome gift. What an amazing gift that the Creator of the universe, who throughout history has created billions and billions of people, still wants to hear from you. He longs to hear your voice and see you humble yourself before Him. He desires your friendship and your adoration. He cares about your needs. He feels your pain. He hears every word you speak.

The fact that God has the supernatural ability to hear all who speak to Him at any given time is incomprehensible. Yet it is true. Doesn't the awesome "otherness" of God generate some questions in your mind? Some praise in your heart? Some outward demonstration in your body?

Then show Him. Make your prayer life a ceaseless function of your body, mind, and heart. Let your prayers flow as frequently and comfortably as your breath. "Be cheerful no matter what; pray all the time; thank God no matter what happens. This is the way God wants you who belong to Christ Jesus to live" (1 Thessalonians 5:16–18 MSG).

Prayer for Abiding

"When I think of the wisdom and scope of God's plan, I fall to my knees and pray to the Father, the Creator of everything in heaven and on earth. I pray that from his glorious, unlimited resources he will give you mighty inner strength through his Holy Spirit. And I pray that Christ will be more and more at home in your hearts as you trust in him. May your roots go down deep into the soil of God's marvelous love. And may you have the power to understand, as all God's people should, how wide, how long, how high, and how deep his love really is. May you experience the love of Christ, though it is so great you will never fully understand it. Then you will be filled with the fullness of life and power that comes from God" (Ephesians 3:14–19).

Part 4

Application

chapter 10

Creating a Flow
(Linking the Postures)

CREATING FLOW IN YOUR PRACTICE INVOLVES LINKING POSTURES TOGETHER FLUIDLY. The melding of the body's movements and the mind's thoughts allows you to keep your concentration more focused during the practice. Adding the Christ-centered intention allows you to enjoy a sort of meditation-in-motion throughout the session.

Baron Baptiste, in his book *Journey into Power*, describes flow as "the absence of resistance. When you bring flow into your practice, you let go into the movements and create a liquid quality that inspires deep release. It allows you to build magnificent momentum and heat and to move through your practice in an effortless, seamless manner. Flow encourages meditation-in-motion: When you ride the flow like a wave, it moves you out of your head and into the body and the present moment."[1]

Linking the postures creates a more energetic and dynamic practice that contributes to weight control and cardiovascular health. The heat that is generated by such a practice increases your flexibility and range of motion, while forcing you to pay deliberate attention to your breath.

I have included several flows as suggestions for sequencing your postures together. Remember that these are only suggestions, and you may decide to make changes, additions, or substitutions as it suits you, your body, your schedule, or your temperament on any given day.

After you have thoughtfully prepared your environment for a quiet, reflective practice session, make sure you have the proper tools at hand: your mat; a blanket, block, or bolster; possibly a strap; and your Bible. Be certain that you are beginning every yoga session with attention to and control of the breath. Make an assessment of your body and mind's health for the day and your intention for the session. As you set your intention, have ready the method by which you plan to focus your thoughts—using the breath of prayer, an affirmation of faith, or quiet preparation for meditation. From there, have in mind how you plan to use your meditation time. Have your Bible open to the scripture you have selected if you plan to "wash yourself in the Word." Have your symbol or object ready if you plan to use it as an aid in visualization.

In other words, to get full enjoyment and spiritual benefit from the session, take a few minutes to prepare and plan before you begin. Doing so will keep you from interrupting the flow of your body and the focus of your mind.

After noticing your breath and setting your intention, take a few moments to limber up. Pay attention to areas of the body that are particularly tight or sensitive. Spend about five to ten minutes preparing your body before moving on to more vigorous postures.

Next, you should choose which warm-up flow you plan to use for the day, either the low-intensity flow or the high-intensity flow. I have included those sequences here as a quick reminder of the postures. Complete at least four cycles of the selected warm-up flow (two on each side) before moving on to the standing postures. Do as many repetitions of the warm-ups as you feel are necessary to begin heating your body as preparation for the rest of the session.

As you choose a flow of postures, keep the pace of your movements correlating with the pace of your breath. Start slowly, noticing how your body reacts to each posture. Remember that your growth doesn't usually happen by just getting into a posture, but by staying there until you find your body releases into the position more comfortably. Be certain that you are making whatever modifications are necessary to practice safely. A good rule of thumb is to allow your body to feel the discomfort of a stretch but not pain. If you ever feel sharp or throbbing pain in a position, carefully release the position and choose the modification or move to the next posture in the sequence.

Building strength and stamina takes time, so don't be discouraged if you have to start more slowly than you had hoped. The postures will flow more smoothly as your body becomes accustomed to them and you are better able to correlate your movements and your breath.

Be persistent. Enjoy the struggle. Be assured that the struggle results in growth.

Low-Intensity Warm-Up Flow

The warm-up flow is designed to build heat. So, once you are familiar with the postures, you may choose to flow through the positions more quickly by moving on each inhale and each exhale.

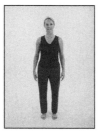

Mountain 4.20

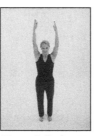

Mountain Peak 4.21
(Inhale)

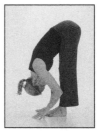

Forward Fold 4.22
(Exhale)

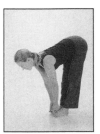

Halfway Lift 4.23
(Inhale)

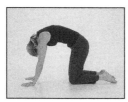

Roll the Back Up 4.24
(Exhale)

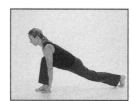

Roll the Back Down 4.25
(Inhale)

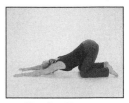

Kneeling-Dog 4.28
(Exhale)

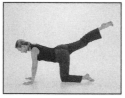

Tabletop Leg Lift 4.29
(Inhale)

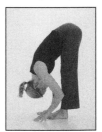

Lunge 4.30
(Exhale)

Standing Forward Fold 4.22
(Inhale—feet together,
Exhale—fold)

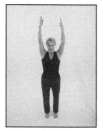

Mountain Peak 4.21
(Inhale)

Follow flow through to the other leg, then repeat at least one more time on each leg.

High-Intensity Warm-Up Flow

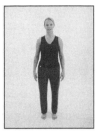

Mountain 4.20

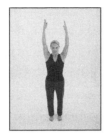

Mountain Peak 4.21
(Inhale)

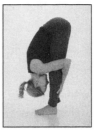

Forward Fold 4.22
(Exhale)

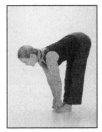

Halfway Lift 4.23
(Inhale)

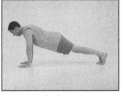

Plank 4.32
(Exhale)

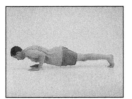

Low Plank 4.33
(Continue Exhale)

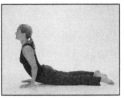

Cobra 4.34
(Inhale)

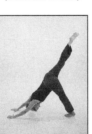

Down Dog 4.27
(Exhale)

Down Dog Leg Lift 4.36
(Inhale)

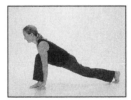

Lunge 4.30
(Exhale)

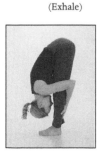

Forward Fold
(Inhale—feet together,
Exhale—fold)

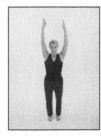

Mountain Peak
(Inhale)

*Again, remember to follow the flow
through to the other leg, and then repeat it
on each leg at least one more time.*

Energizing Flow

This flow, which is relatively high-intensity, is designed to get you up and moving. Most of the postures will allow the body to energize rapidly while working on strength, balance, and mobility. Hold each posture for at least four to five breaths—more as your practice progresses. Postures from the warm-up flow are included to transition you to from one posture series to the next. You may choose to flow through the transitional postures without holding them, but instead moving on each inhale and each exhale.

Remember that you can modify this or any flow to accommodate the level at which you want or need to work. Notice various modifications are offered in the instruction chapter for most of these poses. Also, note that the transition postures are ones used in the high-intensity warm-up flow and can be changed to reflect the postures in the low-intensity warm-up flow. This session should take about one hour to complete, plus time for meditation.

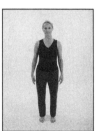
Mountain 4.20

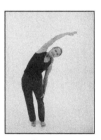
Side Lean 6.5
(both sides)

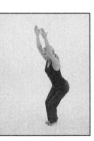
Chair 6.1

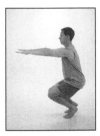
Tiptoe Chair 5.13

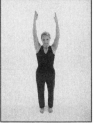
Mountain Peak 4.21

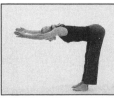
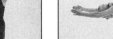
Strong Half Fold 6.3

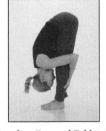
Standing Forward Fold 4.22

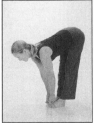
Halfway Lift 4.23

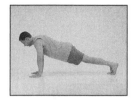

Plank 4.32

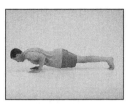

Low Plank 4.33

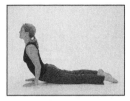

Cobra 4.34

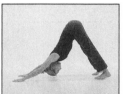

Down Dog 4.27

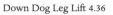

Down Dog Leg Lift 4.36

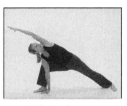

Lunge 4.30

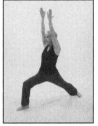

Warrior I 6.12

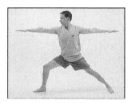

Warrior II 6.13

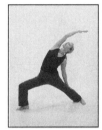

Reverse Warrior 6.14

Side Angle 6.21

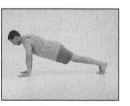

Plank 4.32

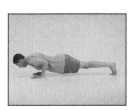

Low Plank 4.33

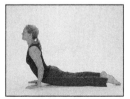

Cobra 4.34

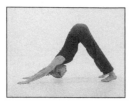

Down Dog 4.27
*Raise left leg and follow sequence
through again to Down Dog

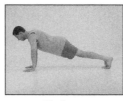

Plank 4.32

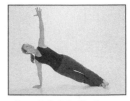

Open Left Side Plank 6.29

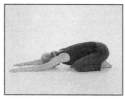

Plank 4.32
*Move left hand center for Right
Side Plank. Return to Plank

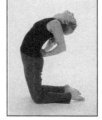

Low Plank 4.33

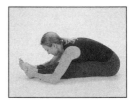

Cobra 4.34

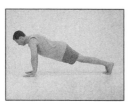

Child's Pose 4.26

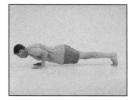

Camel 7.18

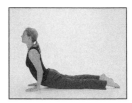

Seated Forward Bend 7.2

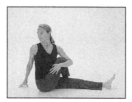

Seated Spinal Twist 7.6
(both sides)

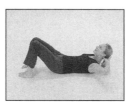

Star Gazer 7.43

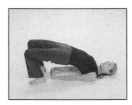

Bridge 7.34

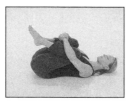

Hugging the Knees 8.1

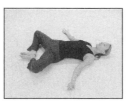

Supine Butterfly 8.4

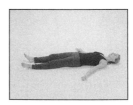

Corpse 8.6

Strength-Focused Flow

This flow still incorporates elements of balance and flexibility but is focused more heavily on developing strength throughout the body. It is best to practice strength flows every other day in order to give the muscles a chance to rest. Alternating days with a more restorative flow will provide a safe and effective practice. Remember to hold postures for at least four to five breaths—longer if possible. You can flow through transitional postures, however, with each inhale and exhale. Expect this flow to take about one hour plus meditation time.

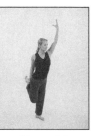

Mountain 4.20

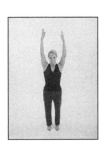

Side Lean 6.5
(both sides)

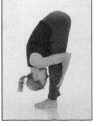

Sanding Leg Raise 5.1
Left Leg

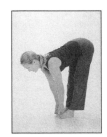

Dancer 5.8
Left Leg

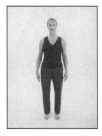

Mountain Peak 4.21

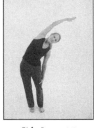

Standing Forward Fold 4.22

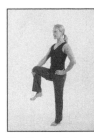

Mountain 4.20

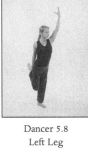

Standing Leg Raise 5.1
Right Leg

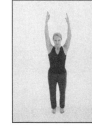

Dancer 5.8
Right Leg

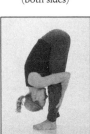

Mountain Peak 4.21

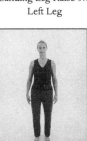

Standing Forward Fold 4.22

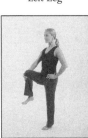

Halfway Lift 4.23

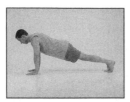

Plank 4.32

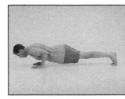

Low Plank 4.33

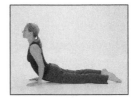

Cobra 4.34

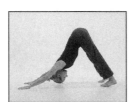

Down Dog 4.27

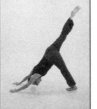

Down Dog Leg Lift 4.36

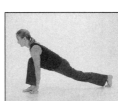

Lunge 4.30

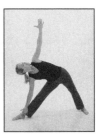

Triangle 6.15b

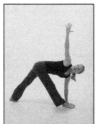

Reverse Triangle 6.15

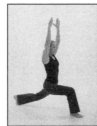

Crescent 6.24

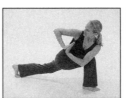

Revolving Crecent 6.26

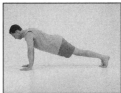

Plank 4.32

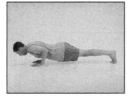

Low Plank 4.33

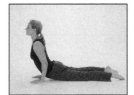

Cobra 4.34

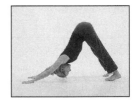

Down Dog 4.27
(lift left leg and follow
sequence through on
other leg to Down Dog.)

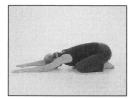

Child's Pose 4.26

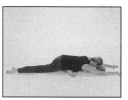

Pigeon 7.26
(both sides)

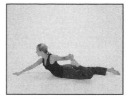

Half-Bow 7.29
(both sides)

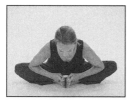

Butterfly 7.10

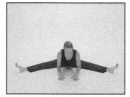

Straddle Forward Fold 7.13

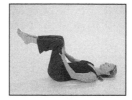

Opposing Resistance 7.46

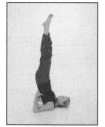

Shoulder Stand 7.48

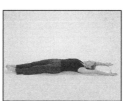

Total Body Reach 8.5

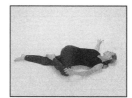

Lying Spinal Twist 8.2
(both sides)

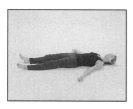

Corpse 8.6

Stretch-Focused Flow

A flow that focuses more heavily on stretching and mobility is safe to practice every day. Make sure you are using your breath to create length and space (on the inhalation) and resting into that space (on the exhalation). Move to the point of challenging your muscles but not causing pain. Pain is your body screaming to you, "You've gone too far!" Listen to your body's cues. This flow should take approximately forty-five minutes to complete, plus meditation time. However, I would suggest that you make it an hour by challenging yourself to hold the postures beyond the usual four to five breaths.

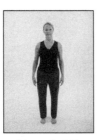

Mountain 4.20

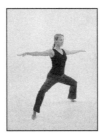

Tiptoe Straddle 5.14

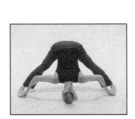

Standing Straddle Fold 6.6

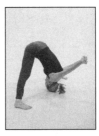

Standing Straddle with arms overhead 6.8

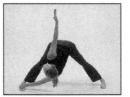

Standing Straddle with twist 6.9

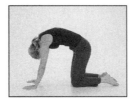

Roll the Back Up 4.24

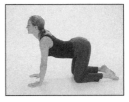

Roll the Back Down 4.25

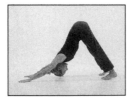

Down Dog 4.27

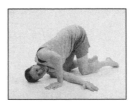

Thread the Needle 7.23
(both sides)

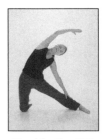

Kneel for Gate 7.21
(both sides)

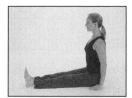

Staff 7.1

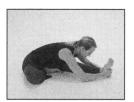

Bent Knee Seated Forward Fold 7.4
(both sides)

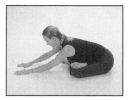

Double Pigeon 7.15
(both sides)

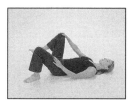

Curl with Butterfly Legs 7.45

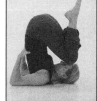

Candlestick 7.50

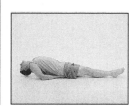

Fish 7.52

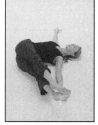

Revolving Legs 7.41
(both sides)

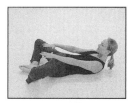

Lying Knee Circles 8.3
(both sides)

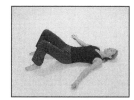

Knees Raised 8.7

Restorative Flow

For a restorative flow, postures should feel like gentle massage for the body. Move more slowly, holding postures about ten breaths, rather than the usual four to five. As you remain in the posture longer, try to notice how your body responds. You should find more openness and movement as you remain in the pose. If instead you feel stuck and uncomfortable, try taking deeper, more intentional diaphragmatic breaths to create more space. This session will take approximately one hour plus time for meditation.

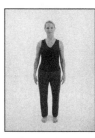
Mountain 4.20

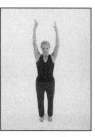
Mountain Peak 4.21

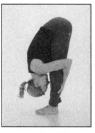
Forward Fold 4.22

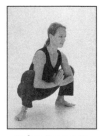
Indian Squat 6.31

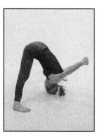
Standing Straddle 6.8
with arms overhead

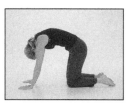
Back up 4.24

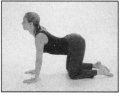
Back down 4.25
(set of 10)

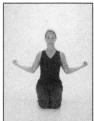
Blade 7.9

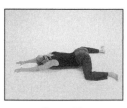
Frog 7.32

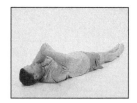
Lying Shoulder Reach 7.37b
(both sides)

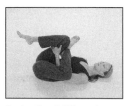
Supine Reach Through 7.39
(both sides)

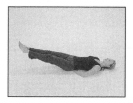

Descending Legs 7.44

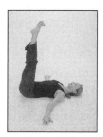

Legs Up the Wall 7.47

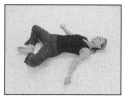

Supine Buttefly 8.4

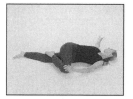

Lying Spinal Twist 8.2

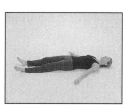

Corpse 8.6

Short Session

Try to give yourself at least an hour to practice if at all possible. However, occasionally you may find that you don't have time to follow a complete session. To create a short session, notice what areas need the most attention, and choose postures that would release, open, or strengthen those areas.

The following is a shorter flow that incorporates most primary target areas. Remember to leave time for relaxation and meditation, even if it is abbreviated. This session should take about thirty minutes plus meditation.

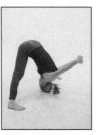
Mountain 4.20

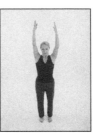
Chair 6.1

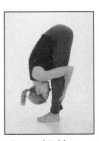
Tree 5.5
(both sides)

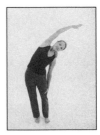
Side Lean 6.5
(both side)

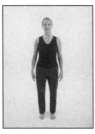
Standing Straddle with
Arms Overhead 6.8

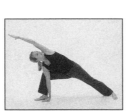
Side Angle 6.21
(both sides)

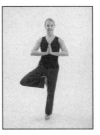
Mountain Peak 4.21

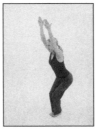
Forward Fold 4.22

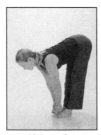
Halfway Lift 4.23

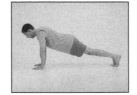
Plank 4.32

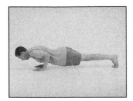
Low Plank 4.33

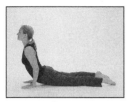

Cobra 4.34

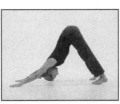

Down Dog 4.27

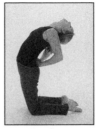

Camel 7.18

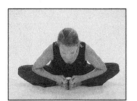

Butterfly 7.10

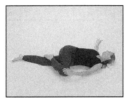

Lying Spinal Twist 8.2
(both sides)

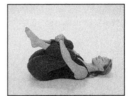

Hugging the Knees 8.1

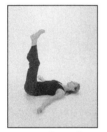

Legs Up the Wall 8.8

chapter 11

Involving Your Children

I ABSOLUTELY LOVE BEING A PARENT. BUT IF YOU'RE LIKE ME, YOU OFTEN HAVE TO BE creative in getting your children to respond with obedience. When my boys were younger (and still occasionally) I would play games with them in order to coax them into the behavior I desired.

If I had errands to run and they really despised the idea of getting into the car, we turned it into a "wild goose chase." The boys seldom realized we were making stops that Mom needed to make, because we were following their directions all over town. If I needed to enter a store that wasn't child-friendly, we played "hands in your pockets." After a while, they would realize Mom's plan of keeping them from breaking the store's finer things, but for a long time it was just another competition to outlast the brother.

My favorite was the one most appropriately used on car trips. Greg and I usually decided it was time to play this game when the noise level and activity in the back seat had reached a fever pitch. You probably know this one. It's called the "mum game," the object of which was to keep the boys as quiet as possible for as long as possible. Of course, this game was a parent favorite, but never one really embraced by my children.

The bottom line is that children really don't see the value of silence. They have questions to ask, experiences to recount, and if all else fails, lots of giggling to do. My sister and I used to giggle so hard in church that our pew would be shaking. My mom would reach over and give the closest one (usually me) a pinch that would hurt for days.

My best friend, Lisa, and I would giggle so hard in class that we once slid out of our desks onto the floor. There was so much giggling going on that often we would have to be separated in class, until eventually the teachers agreed we shouldn't have any more classes together. I couldn't begin to explain what was so funny or why it was the most inappropriate times that set off the frenzy of giggling. But it seldom failed to happen.

It often takes maturity and life experience to understand the value of stillness and quiet. What kind of difference could it make in the life of your child to begin to instill a framework for it now? Whether your child is three or thirteen, you have an opportunity to teach them the fundamentals for creating a restful spirit. That doesn't mean the giggling stops or the questions cease. Those times, though sometimes frustrating, show the beautiful heart of our children and should be allowed to continue whenever appropriate. Instead we could teach them the basics of keeping their bodies healthy while nurturing and equipping their hearts and minds. Statistics indicate that our children are missing these essential ingredients to maintaining a healthy lifestyle.

Not convinced that there is a problem? Check out these statistics:

○ Approximately 30.3 percent of children (ages 6 to 11) are overweight, and 15.3 percent are obese, a higher rate than ever before.

○ Today's youth are considered the most inactive in history.

○ Once considered adult conditions, children are now showing a rise in type 2 diabetes, hypertension, asthma, and orthopedic complications.

○ As many as 3 percent of children and 8 percent of adolescents suffer from depression.

○ A large-scale study by MECA of 9- to 17-year-olds showed that as many as 13 percent of young people had an anxiety disorder in a year.

○ Attention Deficit Hyperactivity Disorder (ADHD) is estimated to affect 3 to 5 percent of school-age children.[1]

Furthermore, our children are exposed to a kind of peer pressure that exceeds that of previous generations. To withstand such pressure, they have to be stronger in spirit and firmer in resolve of their faith than ever before. We have to take our children beyond the stories of the Bible to a faith that guides and instructs them. We have to challenge them to be different, to stand apart for what they believe. We have to teach them to proudly lift the name of Jesus, without fear of embarrassment or ridicule.

In order to do this, we first must create a life with enough margin to spend the necessary time with our children. Second, we must allow enough margin in our children's schedules that they can develop teachable, restful, and listening spirits. Since they model our behavior (unless they are teenagers; then they model the antithesis of our behavior!) we have to first set the example for creating spiritual health.

Begin to model spiritual health by letting your children see you pray, meditate, and listen to God. Let them see you prioritize your Christ-centered yoga practice, getting on the mat on a regular basis. Let them, ultimately, see the change that happens as you feel better in your skin, find contentment with where you are, enjoy God's peace from being in His presence, and make adjustments as you hear God speak into your heart.

Embrace Your Differences

The yoga practice I've described in the previous chapters is completely safe and effective for children as well as adults. However, that doesn't always mean it is practical for children, especially when they are first beginning to practice.

Energy Level

One of the most obvious ways in which a child's practice is different from an adult's is the level of energy. Even the most active adult has a hard time matching the boundless energy of a child. (Put them in a room, telling them they are going to move slowly and quietly and see the energy level rise even more!)

Therefore, the first step in developing a successful child's yoga practice is to find an outlet for that energy before you begin the actual postures. Develop a routine of practicing after some aerobic (code word for "exhausting") activity. The more energy they expend, the better. Try setting up a schedule of running around the block, circling around the house, or chasing the dog before you begin. You can have the child jump rope or do jumping jacks . . . . just get him or her breathing hard before you begin. Set a general timetable of five to twenty minutes of pre-yoga aerobic activity, depending on the age of your child and his or her overall energy level for the day.

Allow them to do their aerobic activity outside of the yoga practice space. Make the yoga space the place where they are always quiet and attentive. Never ask your child to practice where other distractions are present, such as TV or other children playing. Think about creating their environment to be at least as restful as your own practice space.

Rhythm

A child's practice should still move slowly and deliberately, following the pattern of the breath, just like an adult's practice. However, you may have more success in keeping your child interested and engaged if you include some postures that move rhythmically. By rhythmically, I don't mean following the rhythm of the music, but instead following the rhythm of each part of the breath.

For example, notice the Woodchop posture (figure 11.3) or Spinning Swings (figure 11.5). Instead of getting into the posture and holding for five or more breaths, the posture is moving on each inhale and moving on each exhale. This type of rhythmic posture is perfect for those who struggle with focus and attention. If this works for your child, try adapting other postures to move in this way. For example, he or she may get into Chair on an exhale and stand on the following inhale. Continue for five to ten repetitions as your child slowly sits (exhale) and stands (inhale).

As your child's practice develops, holding the posture will become easier. But for now, work with your child's attention level and abilities. Progress to holding only after you are able to keep your child's attention with the rhythmic movements. Moving also makes it fun. Since most children cannot (or will not) appreciate the value of the practice for its health and spiritual benefits just yet, making it fun will keep them coming back for more.

Imagination

Another key to keeping your child's focus during practice is to allow your child to use his or her imagination. A child's imagination is so refreshingly uninhibited and creative. Capitalizing on that creativity will allow your child to understand the postures more thoroughly and remember the postures more readily.

You will notice that each of the posture descriptions in this chapter will include some images your child can connect with the pose. Feel free to create new images to accompany the postures if there is something that more easily connects with your child. The idea is simply to allow your child to feel a part of the movement, not just do it because Mom or Dad said to. For example, if your child is doing Lion pose, let him or her *be* the lion. Let's hear the roar! Let's see those teeth! Make it fun. Be a little silly.

Not only will you and your child have a great time using your imagination as you learn the poses, but you will also see your child respond to the positions more actively and enthusiastically. In addition, you will find that using this expressive technique will help your child commit these poses to memory, which helps develop certain cognitive skills.

Try the following visualization as the foundation pose for every yoga session with your child. Express to your child that this is also his or her foundation for a life in Christ. Be expressive as you describe each piece of armor. Let your child fully visualize how it feels to wear each one.

Visualization

Stand in Mountain pose and visualize yourself in the body armor of Christ from Ephesians 6:10–18.

1. Shoes of peace that come from the Good News so that you will be
   fully prepared (firm footing through both feet).
2. Sturdy belt of truth to stand your ground (firm belly).

3. Faith as your shield to stop the fiery arrows aimed at you by Satan (strong chest).

4. Salvation as your helmet (head resting on top of shoulders, with the face relaxed).

5. Sword of the Spirit, which is the Word of God (repetition of your Breath Prayer—your focus).

Make the Connection

Your child's practice should follow the same general sequence as your adult practice, with the exception of the aerobic activity that will precede your child's yoga postures. Start by noticing the breath and affirming your purpose. Make the spiritual connection with your child regarding each of these aspects, but do so in a way that relates to their level of understanding. Remind them that God gave them each breath that they take and that breath is what gives life to the body. Give them purpose to the practice by sharing a short verse that they can memorize with the breath, such as "I love you, God—you make me strong" (Psalm 18:1 MSG) or "Train me, God, to walk straight" (Psalm 86:11 MSG). Try to express how with this breath of prayer they are attempting to reset their thoughts to this one idea. Let them say it aloud so that it becomes more real, and their minds will not wander.

Next, have your child flow through several warm-ups. Let him or her get used to these warm-up postures until he or she can flow through with ease. Let your child perform as many repetitions as he or she would like, all the while keeping his or her thoughts focused on the breath of prayer. Let your child know that the main function of the warm-up is to prepare the body (by building heat to make the muscles more subtle) and preparing the heart and mind (by burning away distractions and worries that crowd the mind and keep the heart from hearing and knowing God).

After your child is warmed up, start with balance postures. Always let your child develop confidence in balance by working with the wall or a chair. Normally, children struggle much more with balance than they do strength or flexibility. This is usually more a function of attention than misalignment. Therefore, allow them to work on their focus by having a very defined focal point at which they can gaze. Keep reminding your child to keep the eyes focused on that point at all times during the balance posture. Challenge your child to move away from the wall only as he or she develops more confidence and focus with the postures. If focus continues to be an issue with your child, always precede any balance posture with the Thumb Focus exercise (figure 11.10, described on pg. 196).

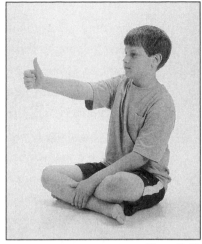

Figure 11.10

Make the connection with your child that God is the solid foundation that keeps us balanced. Help your child become aware that in the midst of all the competing distractions, God is the constant, calming, steady rhythm by which we can set our lives.

From here let your child build strength and heat with some standing postures. Warrior postures are usually fun and empowering for children. Help your child notice the strength he or she begins to develop in these postures, but make the connection that true strength comes only from God. Encourage your child to visualize that each breath that he or she takes is actually the empowering of the Holy Spirit. Remind your child that he or she is totally dependent on Him.

I know this idea of dependency is contrary to popular opinion in raising our children. Many "experts" will advise parents to empower their children, making them independent and self-sufficient. Perhaps this line of thinking is why many young adults today reject God, feeling that they are self-made and need no one but themselves. Children need to understand at an early age that while self-esteem is important, their real power and purpose come only from knowing God and believing in Jesus as their Savior. Why should we expect them to mature into understanding their dependency on God if we have ingrained in them a self-sufficiency to accomplish all things on their own power?

Move from strength to stretching with your child as you come to the mat for floor postures. For most children, a huge hurdle in this segment will be learning to let go and relax into the pose. Remind your child continually to keep the breath flowing. Point out, with each breath, how the exhale is allowing him or her to feel more comfortable in the posture. Even exaggerate the movement from inhale (lengthening) to exhale (relaxing deeper) until your child understands the concept of how to get movement with the breath.

Talk about freedom here. Start by pointing out the freedom we experience from the immediate struggle in yoga postures by simply relaxing and letting go. Make the connection that freedom in Christ is much the same: When we release all our struggles to the One who died for us we can experience a life of freedom. We no longer have to worry about what our peers think of us, if we have the right shoes, if we have the right clothes, or if we are willing to give in to whatever behavior is popular at the moment. We don't have to worry about trends and fads, because our God is constant, unchanging, and always available. He never divorces us, moves away, or gets a new best friend. Relate to your child using circumstances and experiences that are familiar and age-appropriate.

Finally, move into rest and relaxation with your child. Here is your biggest challenge in developing your child's practice: persuading your child that being quiet and still is actually good! Since most children do not value silence and stillness, this will be an acquired skill. You will probably need to start with a very short period of stillness and lengthen it as your child develops this skill. Start by allowing your child to lie in any position that feels comfortable to him or her. This may involve curling up on one side or even lying on the stomach with a pillow. Let your child decide what feels like the best position for relaxation.

Have your child take several deep breaths to help relax onto the floor. Make sure his or her eyes are closed, even suggesting a little towel rest over the eyes so he or she won't be tempted to open them. Make sure your child's body is warm and covered. Get rid of any exterior distractions that may still exist. Eliminate as much outside noise as is possible.

Tell your child to let the entire body rest heavily on the floor and to feel as if he or she is "melting" into the mat. Use this opportunity while your child is relaxed and receptive to reinforce the one concept you began with in your breath scripture. Have them say it in their hearts a couple of times. Ask them to quietly pray about what this means to them and their life. Let the thought soak in. Have them visualize how their behavior and attitudes might change to reflect this new understanding. Have them listen to what God is saying to them. Try to guide their thoughts in general, but do so concisely and reverently, so that they can do most of the listening with their hearts and not their ears.

Cultivating a quiet, restful spirit in your children will have lifelong benefits. It will enable them to become less reliant on outside stimuli, such as TV and computer games. It will provide them with a portable stillness that will keep them calm when life becomes chaotic. And finally, creating a spirit of stillness and quiet will teach your children to become God-focused rather than self-focused. It will be an avenue through which your children can learn lifelong prayer habits to develop a closer, more intimate relationship with God.

Add New Postures

While all the postures described in previous chapters are safe for children, they may consider some to be more enjoyable and easier to understand. Choose a flow of postures that makes the practice fun, while still challenging them to go outside their comfort zone. Following are a few additional poses that are a good fit for a child's practice.

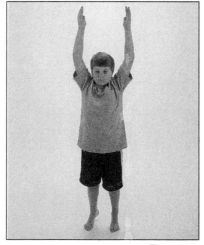

Tiptoe Reach—*lengthens the spine, strengthens the legs, develops balance, encourages focus* (figure 11.1)
1. Start in your firm foundation posture of Mountain pose. Then separate your feet about hip-width apart.
2. Fix your gaze on something stationary that is directly in front of you.
3. On an inhale, raise the arms overhead, pulling up and out through the fingertips.

Figure 11.1

4. On an exhale, make sure your face and shoulders are relaxed.

5. On an inhale, keep the arms overhead and raise up onto the ball of the foot, trying your best to balance there.

6. Slowly lower your heels back to the floor on an exhale.

7. Try to balance up (inhale) and down (exhale) for eight to ten repetitions.

Visualization

Imagine yourself as an astronaut who becomes weightless in space. Ground and balance firmly with the heels down as if standing on Earth. But lift onto the toes to make your body light and weightless as if in space. Keep your gaze focused on the horizon ahead.

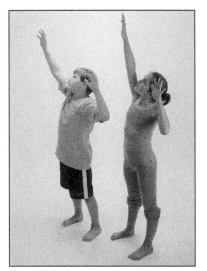

Figure 11.2

One-Arm Reach—*lengthens the side body and back, stretches the shoulder, awakens the body* (figure 11.2)

1. Start again in Mountain pose. Make sure feet are about hip-width apart.

2. On an inhale, raise the arms overhead to reach for the sky.

3. On an exhale, relax your shoulders and face.

4. On an inhale, look up toward your fingertips and raise the right arm higher than the left. Keep both feet grounded.

5. On an exhale, release that side so that both sides are equal again.

6. On the next inhale, reach higher through the left arm. Keep your gaze upward.

7. Alternate reaching with each arm on the inhales for eight to ten repetitions.

Visualization

Imagine you are standing beneath an orange tree, ripe with fruit. With one hand at a time, you are reaching for the juicy orange that is just out of reach. Continue reaching higher and higher to pick the fruit that you desire.

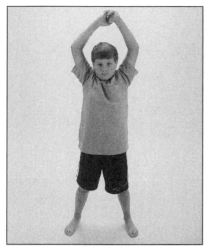

Figure 11.3a

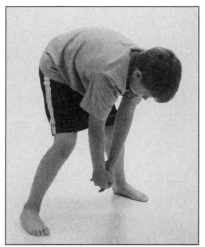

Figure 11.3b

Woodchopper—*wakes up the whole body to fill you with energy, improves circulation, loosens up neck and back*

1. Stand with legs a little more than hip-width apart. Keep the knees slightly bent.

2. Place your hands together as if you are holding the handle of an axe. Make a strong fist.

3. Inhale and raise your fists overhead. (figure 11.3a)

4. On an exhale, bend the knees deeply as you bend at the waist and allow your arms to fall forward and downward. Bend as far as you can as you chop down. (figure 11.3b)

5. Raise up on the inhale, chop down on the exhale for eight to ten repetitions.

6. Increase the energy by breathing more deeply with each chop.

7. As you get loosened up, feel free to swing all the way through the legs.

Visualization

Imagine that you are a lumberjack with lots of work to do. Create enough energy upward with each inhale to help you chop through your log on the exhale. Think about the energy and strength it would take to actually split the log. Stay focused on your work.

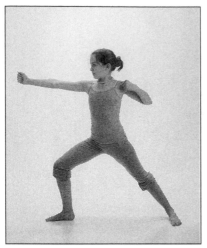

Figure 11.4

Archer—*strengthens the legs, abs, and arms; opens the chest; improves focus* (figure 11.4)

1. Stand with legs wide and spine very tall.

2. Relax your shoulders down, and soften your facial muscles.

3. Turn your right foot to face out and your left foot in about halfway.

4. Bend the right knee, trying to get the thigh parallel to the floor. Don't let the knee push out over the toes, but let it line up over the heel.

5. Keep your hips and chest facing open.

6. On an inhale, bring both arms up to shoulder height over the right leg, with fists facing in toward one another. Look out over your fists.

7. With strong fists, draw the left arm back toward the chest. Keep the right arm straight and extended. Keep the back straight and the shoulder open, not rounded.

8. Keep your gaze fixed forward as you bend the front knee a little more.

9. Breathe deeply with your abs tight for five or more breaths.

10. Change to the other side for the same number of breaths.

Visualization

Imagine that you are a skilled archer aiming at your target. Pretend there is a large bow in your right hand and you are pulling back on the string with your left. Keep your target focused in your line of sight. Think of the strength and stamina required to actually aim, wait patiently, then hit the target.

Spinning Swings—*loosens your arms, back, and waist; energizes the upper body; stabilizes the lower body* (figure 11.5)

1. Stand with your legs a little more than hip-width apart.

2. On an inhale, lengthen your spine upward.

3. On an exhale, relax your shoulders and facial muscles. Engage the abdominals.

4. Keep your breath flowing as you begin turning your upper body from one side to the other. Alternate sides as you let your arms swing freely.

5. Let your head turn as your upper body swings side to side, but keep your feet and hips stationary.

6. Keep the legs strong and hips facing front.

7. Pick up momentum as you move, swinging farther and farther around.

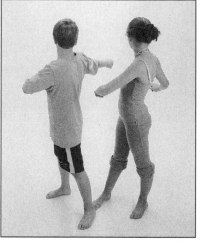

Figure 11.5

Visualization

Imagine the spinning swings ride at the fair. Your body is the base of the ride, strong and stable. Your arms are two of the spinning swings, circling the ride. Make it a fun ride for your passengers with the swings spinning freely.

Rock the Baby—*opens the hip and groin; strengthens abs, back, shoulders, and arms* (figure 11.6)

1. Sit with your legs crossed comfortably, right leg on the top. For more comfort, you may choose to sit on a folded blanket or towel.

2. Keep the right knee bent as you reach down with both hands and grab the leg. Try to hold the leg so that the right foot nestles into the bend of the left elbow and the right arm cradles the right knee.

3. Be very gentle with the knee as you use the arms to draw the leg in and up toward your chest.

4. Keep lengthening up through the spine to keep the back straight.

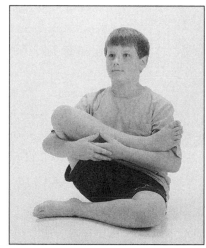

Figure 11.6

5. Once the hip joint and knee feel more comfortable, begin to gently rock your raised leg back and forth in a side-to-side motion.

6. Rock here for about ten breaths before moving to the other leg.

Visualization

Pretend that you are holding a tiny baby in your arms. Rock the baby soothingly and steadily. Keep the baby nestled as close to your body as you can. Remember, babies can sense tension, so breathe deeply to be relaxed as you rock.

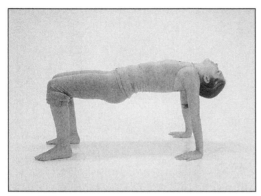

Figure 11.7

Crab—*strengthens the upper body; tones the hips, abs, and thighs; opens the chest and throat; builds core strength* (figure 11.7)

1. Sit with your legs extended in front of you.

2. Bend the knees until the feet are resting flat on the floor. Keep the feet about hip-width apart and parallel.

3. Place your hand behind you with fingers facing toward the feet.

4. Inhale and lift your hips to form a straight line from shoulders to knees.

5. Exhale and let your head rest back gently.

6. Press firmly through the feet and keep the abs engaged.

7. Continue breathing deeply here for five or more breaths.

Visualization

Imagine that you are a sand crab who has wandered far from the hole in the sand in which you live. All around you on the beach are sunbathers and children who would love to catch you. You must remain perfectly still as you wait for them to look the other way so that you can dart quickly back to your hole.

Lion—*releases tension in the face, jaw, and throat* (figure 11.8)

1. Sit with your feet resting under your buttocks. Release your toes so that you are resting on the top of the foot. Place your hands, palms down, on your knees.

2. Inhale and lengthen up through the spine.

3. Exhale and relax the shoulders and face.

4. nhale and energize. On the exhale open your mouth and eyes as wide as they will go. Stick your tongue out as far as you can.

5. Spread your fingers to engage all the way up the arms and look upward from the eyes, but without moving the head.

6. Let your exhale last as long as possible.

7. Relax the tongue, face, arms, and hands on the inhale.

8. Repeat one or two more times until your lungs feel refreshed with new air.

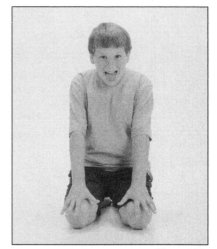

Figure 11.8

Visualization

Imagine that you are the powerful lion, the mighty king of the beasts. Open your mouth wide and let out a ferocious roar as you exhale.

Z Force—*develops core strength, stretches legs and feet, improves posture* (figure 11.9)

1. Kneel on the floor with the knees about hip-width apart.

2. On an exhale, relax your shoulders and facial muscles.

3. On an inhale, lengthen the spine tall and raise the arms out in front of you to be parallel to the floor.

4. Exhale and engage the abs. Let your body lean back at an angle to create a Z shape with the arms, torso, and legs. Don't let your buttocks drop back toward your heels. Keep your hips forward and in a straight line with your spine.

5. Keep the face relaxed and neck calm.

6. Try to maintain strong abs as you breathe deeply here for five or more breaths.

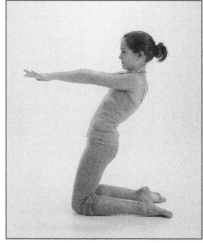

Figure 11.9

Visualization

Pretend that you are driving in a race car so fast that your body is forced backward at an angle. Keep pulling up tall, however, so you can see over the steering wheel. Remember to stay focused and breathing in order to maintain control of the car.

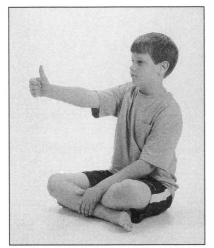

Figure 11.10

Thumb Focus—*improves focus and concentration, calms* (figure 11.10)

1. Sit comfortably with legs crossed or tucked behind you.

2. Extend one arm out in front of you with a loose fist, thumb facing up.

3. Focus your gaze directly onto the thumb and begin deepening your breath.

4. Without changing your gaze, try bringing the thumb forward toward the face (exhale) and outward again (inhale) several times.

5. Keep the arm extended, focusing on the thumb only, for ten or more breaths.

Visualization

Imagine that you are a big-league pitcher who is having some difficulty throwing strikes. Your thumb is the catcher's mitt, and you are trying to eliminate all other distractions so you can focus on the mitt. The screaming crowd begins to blur, the pressure eases, and you feel yourself centering on this one thing.

Create a Flow

Creating a flow to your postures takes on even greater importance in a child's practice. You want your child to learn to pause and breathe while in the pose, but hesitating between postures will allow your child to become distracted and unfocused. Keep things moving to retain your child's attention throughout the session.

Plan a steady rhythm of postures that follows the same general sequence as your adult practice: warm-up, balance, strength, stretch, and rest. Integrate postures described in previous chapters with those in this chapter to create a well-balanced class. Pay attention not only to what movements your child enjoys but also to where your child struggles and needs attention. Design the flow to complement both of these areas.

The following is a sample flow ideal for children. This flow should take thirty to forty-five minutes plus meditation. (Remember that a child's attention span is generally shorter than an adult's, so plan a shorter session and lengthen it as your child is ready.)

Complete the warm-up flow of your choice at least four times (2 on each leg) before beginning this sequece.

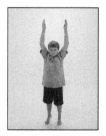

Tip Toe Reach 11.1

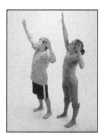

One-Arm Reach 11.2
(both sides)

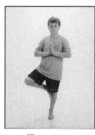

Tree 5.5
(both sides)

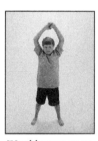

Woodchopper 11.3a

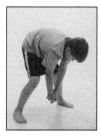

Woodchopper 11.3b

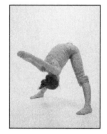

Standing Straddle with
Arms Overhead 6.8

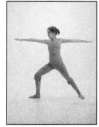

Warrior II 7.13

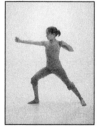

Archer 11.4

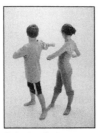

Spinning Swings 11.5
(both sides)

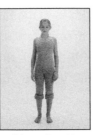

Mountain 4.20

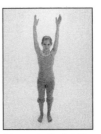

Mountain Peak 4.21

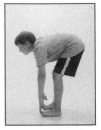

Halfway Lift 4.22

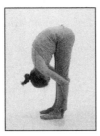

Forward Fold 4.23

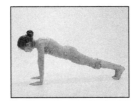

Plank 4.32

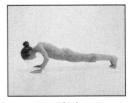

Low Plank 4.33

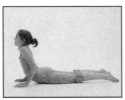

Cobra 4.34

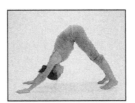

Down Dog 4.27

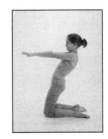

Z Force 11.9

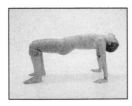

Crab 11.7

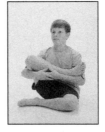

Rock the Baby 11.6
(both sides)

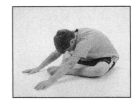

Butterfly 7.10

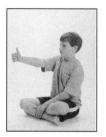

Revolving Legs 7.41

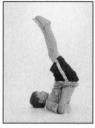

Shoulder Stand 7.48

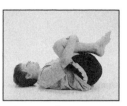

Hugging the Knees 8.1

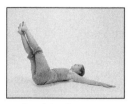

Thumb Focus 11.10

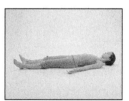

Corpse 8.6

chapter 12

Connecting with a Partner

A BEAUTIFUL WOMAN, WHOM I'LL INTRODUCE TO YOU AS KAREN (NOT HER REAL name), recently began coming to my classes. She is an older woman who lost her husband about a year ago and has no children. She is relatively new to the area, so she has yet to make any close friends and has no family or support system. She is not a Christian, so she has made no church affiliation or relationships. I am so thankful that Karen found our classes because, before she did, she admittedly had virtually no contact with anyone. No one talked to her. No one cared if she woke up each morning. No one touched her. Her health had begun to decline, and she didn't even have transportation to the hospital.

Karen has come alive in her twice-weekly visits to class. She is talkative and engaging, and her health is progressively improving. She shared with me that the interaction she has with us is nourishing to her spirit. And while her belief system has yet to make the change, she is thoughtful and questioning about the Christian emphasis we place on the class. She has also noticed what we have: a love for one another of which she is now a part.

Human contact is more than just enjoyable; it is vital to your well-being. Yet in today's world, we can go days, even weeks, without actually talking to or touching another person. We can correspond with someone via e-mail. We can work from our homes, exercise with a television show, shop online, and have dinner ordered in.

In many ways, modern technology has limited actual human contact. Yet our bodies, minds, and spirits still long for that interaction and touch. A handshake can establish relationship and trust, or an embrace can comfort and calm fears. (Note that if you are in a family with young children, there may be a different need surfacing for you, and that is the need for *less* human contact. But that's another issue entirely!)

We all need healthy relationships, and within those relationships we need a healthy touch. Practicing yoga with a partner, whether it is a spouse, family member, or friend, can be a very positive way to connect and build relationship. It connects people with the element of trust and surrender. It creates an awareness of looking not only to your own needs but also caring about the needs of others. It widens your perspective to move away from a self-centered, "What is this posture doing for me?" mentality and into a cooperative focus as you attempt to remain in sync with your partner.

Physically, a yoga practice that includes some partner postures will challenge you to greater strength and flexibility. It will allow you to move with better posture and alignment. Generally, it will take you to the next level in developing your practice and fine-tuning your poses.

Most of my students are delighted to find we are going to include partner work on any given day. However, there are those who would rather have dental work than work with a partner. They don't like to be touched, and they aren't comfortable touching someone else. Partner yoga may not be preferable for everyone. But there is so much physical and emotional growth that can be achieved that I want to encourage you to give it a try.

Choosing a Partner

The most important factor in choosing a partner is determining with whom you feel comfortable and relaxed. The goal of partner work is not to determine who is the strongest or most flexible, but to assist, support, and work interdependently. If you cannot do so comfortably with your partner, choose a new practice buddy.

It is not necessary for partners to be practicing at the same level. An advanced student can learn much about patience and generosity by working with a beginner. Of course, two more advanced students working together can progress to more difficult postures, but learning something along the way is just as important.

Finding a partner who is similar in height and weight is helpful but not necessary. If you and your partner vary greatly in size, you will simply need to be that much more aware and attuned to what you are doing to make the postures work effectively.

Communication between partners is extremely important. Since you can't feel what your partner is feeling, you must rely on him (or her) to verbalize his limits. Having a clear picture of how far your partner wants to progress in each pose is crucial to both of you remaining safe and healthy. Don't hesitate to calmly tell your partner, "That's enough" or, "I think I can go a little farther." Keep the small talk to a minimum (since it interrupts the breath), but verbalize clearly what you need in each posture to ensure maximum growth with the least risk of injury.

Practicing with the same person regularly is helpful so that you can become more knowledgeable about each of your needs and abilities. Over time, vocalizing your needs may become less necessary as you and your partner are able to recognize each other's body language and personal limits.

Remember that some partner poses will challenge your balance, some your strength, and others your flexibility. Regardless of the posture, your partner needs to be able to experience a level of trust and surrender with you that allows her to relax. You must learn to work together in both self-awareness and partner awareness.

Synchronizing the Breath

Your breath is just as important in partner work as it is in your personal practice. It is still the foundation for all your movement and the ongoing opportunity for you to become both energized and tension-free. It is your personal gift of life from your Creator and the tangible expression of the Holy Spirit within you.

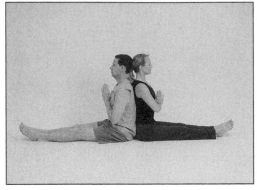

Figure 12.1

Therefore, if partners plan to work interdependently, then the breath must be synchronized to flow together. Try this exercise from *Partner Yoga* to begin coordinating the breath (figure 12.1).[1]

Sit back to back with your legs extended in front of you. Press your back gently against your partner's back until you feel a firm connection along the entire length of the spine. Adjust your posture until you feel that you are equally supported by and supporting your partner. Bring your hands together, with your thumb at the breastbone. Close your eyes and listen to your breath. Feel your ribs rise and fall against your hands. Notice how your back expands and contracts against your partner's.

Begin to notice now how your partner is breathing. Take note of the rate, depth, and sound. Then slowly begin to adjust your breathing pattern to match your partner's. Since it is likely that one of you will have a longer breathing pattern than the other, you will need to meet somewhere in the middle, where you both feel comfortable. Stay here for about five minutes as you breathe together, creating a rhythm and pattern. Stay focused and relaxed as you prepare for practice.

An Expression of Servanthood

Partner work is another opportunity for you to integrate your physical development with your spiritual health. Begin to look at each partner session as a chance to practice servanthood. Consider how you can best assist or support your partner. Become aware of your partner's needs and make them more important than your own. Jesus instructs us to live life with just this attitude in Mark 10:43–45 when He says, "Whoever wants to be a leader among you must be your servant and whoever wants to be first must be the slave of all. For even

I, the Son of Man, came here not to be served but to serve others, and to give my life as a ransom for many."

Jesus, as we've noted, is the ultimate counterculturalist (one of the many reasons I feel He blesses this yoga ministry). He didn't look at society and remark, "Well, this is the way it has always been done." Instead, He turned tradition on its ear by expressing a path to greatness that comes from being a servant. It was a radical thought then, and it's a radical thought now. An amazing thing happens when you begin to serve others, you begin to see the truth about yourself, who you really are.

This is never more evident than when a mission team returns from a trip to an impoverished nation of people they have come to "help." Although great work is usually accomplished during the visit—perhaps a school or a church is built or money is delivered for future projects—yet the overwhelming response by those who attend is that they receive far more than they give. Their lives are enriched not by things or souvenirs of the trip but by relationships and the love that comes from serving.

Living a life of servanthood is one way to enjoy the kingdom of God right now. Begin to notice the needs of others. Consider how you can put those needs above your own. Restructure your life to be a giver and not just a taker. Let God change your perspective so that servanthood and submission are the natural by-products of your gratitude to the ultimate Servant who died for you.

Partner-Assisted Postures

There are two broad types of partner postures: partner-assisted postures, in which you are supporting your partner through the pose, and interdependent postures, in which you are both receiving benefit from the pose at the same time.

The attitude of servanthood can be best demonstrated in partner-assisted work. Your growth during this portion of class comes simply from giving of yourself to your partner. Through your assistance, your partner can achieve better alignment and posture. With your support, your partner can move to depths of greater flexibility and balance. You simply get to be the vehicle through which this growth occurs. (Of course, you will also want to trade places with your partner at some point and be the recipient as well.)

You will need the same items you used in your personal practice, with the addition of a strap. If you don't have a yoga strap, a necktie or scarf can work just as effectively.

Start the session with you and your partner discussing any health issues that might be a factor in your work together. Discuss how you are feeling today and what your overall intention is for this time. Take time to synchronize your breath so that you can move with that rhythm through your postures.

After you have synchronized your breath, face one another, reach out and touch one another, and thank God for the gift of this person. Ask God for healing and protection of your partner. Ask God for direction and guidance in your partner's life. Thank God for bringing you together for the purpose of physical and spiritual growth.

Even if it feels a little awkward at first, pray for your partner anyway. It is a blessing and a comfort to know that someone is praying on your behalf. Let your partner enjoy that blessing, and let it bring you together as practice partners and partners in Christ.

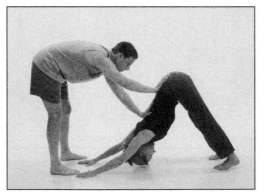

Figure 12.2

Assisted Downward-Facing Dog

As your partner flows through a warm-up flow, help him or her fine-tune the Downward-Facing Dog pose in any of these three ways. In fact, it may be helpful to have your partner flow through three times and you assist him in one of three different ways each time.

1. As your partner lifts the tailbone in Down Dog, place one hand on the upper back and the other on the sacrum.

Press gently up and back to flatten and lengthen the back. Have your partner keep his hands in the same spot without walking them back as you adjust the spine (figure 12.2)

2. As your partner sinks the heels in Down Dog, stand behind the legs and grab the front of the upper thighs (figure 12.3).

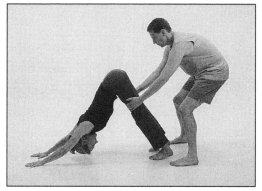

Figure 12.3

Gently pull back on the thighs to create length through the spine and energy through the legs. Again, don't let your partner walk the hands back due to the backward pull from the legs (figure 12.4).

3. As your partner lengthens out from the hands through the shoulders, stand in front and roll the armpits and deltoid muscles inward and slightly downward. Have your partner roll his elbows inward toward one another. This spiraling motion will help protect the shoulders and relieve pressure in the wrists.

Assisted Cobra

As your partner flows through the warm-up, it is also helpful for you to assist in Cobra. Be certain that you are listening carefully to your partner as you assist him in this pose so that you do not run the risk of injuring your partner's shoulders. Let your partner flow through one or two warm-ups before attempting to assist in Cobra to allow adequate stretching and lubricating of the back (figure 12.4).

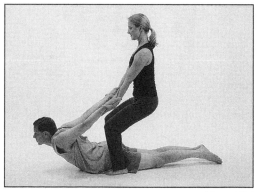

Figure 12.4

1. As your partner gets ready to lift into Cobra, stand over him with your legs on either side of his hips.

2. Bend your knees so that your partner can reach back and you are able to take hold of his wrists in a firm hold.

3. Have your partner relax his shoulders down away from the ears and lengthen the spine.

4. Slowly begin to stand straighter as you hold your partner's wrists. This will allow him to lift his torso off the mat, strengthening the lower back and opening the chest and shoulders.

5. As he lifts, have your partner tuck the tailbone downward, press the hips forward, and create a gentle arc.

6. Let your partner tell you how high to lift and how long he feels comfortable staying in this assisted position.

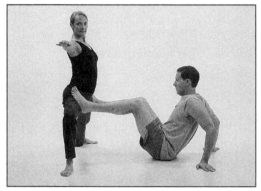

Figure 12.5

Assisted Warrior II

Use assisted Warrior II as an opportunity to realize how the posture should feel with proper alignment. Notice how far your usual Warrior pose is from this ideal. Try to stay long enough in the assisted posture to create some muscle memory for the legs, hips, and back (figure 12.5).

1. Find a length of empty wall space so that your partner can assume Warrior II with his back against the wall. Line the back, heel, both shoulders, and both hips against the wall. Line up the front heel with the back arch.

2. Sit on the floor in front of your partner. Place your feet on his inner thighs, and gently begin to roll the thighs outward and upward.

3. Adjust your partner slowly until the hips are both as close to the wall as is possible for your partner. Make sure that he is keeping the bent leg at a 90-degree angle with the knee directly over the heel.

4. Have your partner keep his arms extended outward and parallel to the floor. Remind him to keep lengthening the spine upward by moving the ribcage away from the hips and relaxing the shoulders downward.

5. Stay here until your partner begins to develop some muscle memory, and then switch to the other leg.

Assisted Preparation for Triangle

Often in Triangle, students want to move much farther than their bodies are actually ready to go. Rather than create misalignment (or worse yet, an injury), try this assisted pose to establish proper posture and more appropriate movement (figure 12.6).

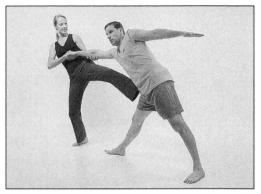

Figure 12.6

1. Have your partner stand tall with his legs in position for Triangle pose. Have him extend his arms outward, with shoulders relaxed.

2. Stand in front of your partner's extended leg, about one to two feet away from his toes.

3. Balance on one leg as you place the other foot in your partner's hip crease.

4. Hold your partner's extended arm, pulling gently forward on the arm as you push gently back on the hip crease. Have your partner lean outward with the arm while keeping the legs the same.

5. Create as much of a fold at the hip as you can so your partner can lengthen the spine and both sides of the body.

6. Stay here long enough to create some muscle memory for your partner. Then release and let him reach down for his foot, his ankle, a block, or the floor, depending on how much space was created.

7. Assist your partner on the other leg.

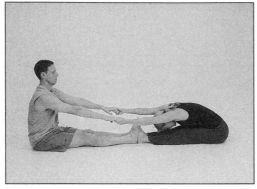

Figure 12.7

Assisted Seated Forward Fold

In this fold, you should always feel a little outward movement with each inhale and a little downward movement with each exhale. However, students will often feel "stuck" in one spot and need a little assistance to relax into more movement. Remember that the breath, and not your partner's assistance, should be the main force in creating more movement.

There are actually a couple of different ways to assist your partner in this position, with the most basic being simply resting your hands gently on your partner's back and helping him or her move downward on each exhale. For greater assistance, try the following assisted posture (figure 12.7).

1. Both you and your partner should be sitting on the floor, with your legs extended and the bottoms of your feet resting against your partner's.

2. On an inhale, have your partner lengthen his spine and reach his arms overhead to lengthen both sides of the body as well.

3. On an exhale, have your partner hinge at the hips, bend forward, and reach out for his toes. As he does, reach out for your partner's arms and hold him firmly around the wrists.

4. Keeping your back as straight as possible, gently pull on your partner's arms to guide him out and over his legs. Try to create as much length in his back as is possible at this time.

5. Make sure both of your are keeping your legs straight and necks relaxed.

6. See if a little more movement can be created with each breath.

Assisted Butterfly

Trying to maintain a long, tall back is one of the greatest challenges of the Butterfly pose. Try this assisted pose to correct your posture and gain greater flexibility (figure 12.8)

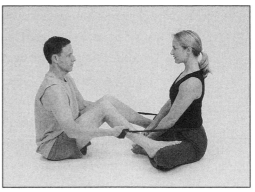

Figure 12.8

1. Have your partner sit on a mat or folded blanket with the soles of the feet together. Your partner should be holding his big toes with the back lifting tall and the knees relaxing down.

2. Sit on the floor facing your partner and wrap a strap around his lower back, right above the sacrum.

3. At the same time, rest your feet on your partner's shins to encourage the hips to open and the knees to relax down.

4. Hold the ends of the strap in each hand to draw your partner's back to an even taller posture by pulling the strap gently toward yourself.

5. Notice how much your partner's spine lengthens and his knees relax down as you encourage him with the strap and the feet. Stay here until your partner begins to feel some muscle memory, and then release and let him hinge and fold his chest toward his feet in Butterfly.

Assisted Fish

Try this assisted posture to achieve more opening in the chest and better preparation for backbends. Verbalize to your partner how you are feeling *before* you feel you've gone too far (figure 12.9).

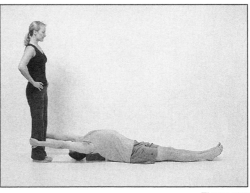

Figure 12.9

1. Have your partner lie on his back on the mat. Have him lift into Fish pose with the support of a rolled blanket or a block placed right under the sternum. Your partner's head should relax off the end of the blanket or block comfortably.

2. Make sure your partner is lifting through the breastbone and lengthening out from the hips through the feet.

3. Stand behind your partner so that your feet are about arms-length behind your partner's head.

4. Have your partner reach the arms overhead, rolling the armpits and deltoid muscles toward one another.

5. Let your partner grab your shins. As the extension gets more comfortable, take little steps backward to challenge him more.

6. Stay in this challenging position as long as you can still breathe comfortably.

Interdependent Partner Postures

Interdependent postures allow you and your partner to feel benefits of the pose at the same time. This makes it even more vital that you communicate with your partner regarding how you are feeling. Be sensitive not only to what you are feeling in your body, but what feelings are being created in your partner's body at the same time. Be patient and understanding with your partner, especially if he is working at a different level from yours. Remember that benefit will come from both serving and being served.

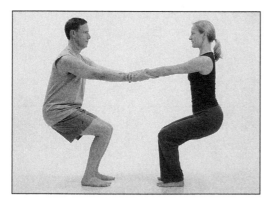

Figure 12.10

Double Chair

This partner posture will allow you to build body heat while challenging your strength and balance. Begin to establish trust as you lower together (figure 12.10).

1. Face one another in Mountain pose as you stand about one to two feet apart.

2. Reach out and loosely grab one another's upper arms.

3. Keep the belly firm and the back tall as you slowly sit back into Chair position. As you sit back, let your hands slide down

your partner's arms until you are linking at the wrists.

4. Try to sit back far enough that your knees are over your ankles and your thighs are parallel to the ground.

5. Keep the face and shoulders relaxed and your gaze focused on one another.

6. Stay here for five or more breaths as you work to build trust with your partner.

7. Continue to maintain balance as you lift back up slowly.

Double Side Lean

Working with a partner for standing postures will definitely challenge your balance and stability. Use this posture to open the side of the body and create awareness of the alignment in your hip and spine (figure 12.11).

1. Stand side by side with your partner, about three feet apart.

2. Let the inside hands connect in a low angle, with the palms pressing against one another. (Note that the partner with the shorter limbs should have the front hand pressing back, and the longer-limbed partner should have the back hand with the palm pressing forward.)

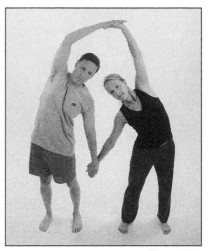

Figure 12.11

3.Lengthen up through the spine, relax the shoulders and face, and firm the belly.

4. On an inhale, raise the outside arms up and connect them overhead at the palms. Press the palms against one another. (Again, the shorter limb is on the bottom pressing up, and the longer is on the top pressing down.)

5. Allow the hips to push slightly out away from each other, but keep the spine long and belly firm as you press the palms firmly together.

6. Feel the side of the body lengthen as you hold at least five breaths before moving to the other side.

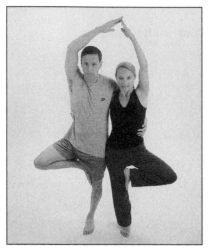

Figure 12.12

Double Tree

Work on stabilizing with your partner in this balance pose. Synchronized breathing and proper posture will make this one a breeze (figure 12.12).

1. Stand side by side with your bodies hip to hip. Your inside foot will end up about eight to twelve inches away from your partner's.

2. Hold each other around the waist until you feel stabilized and balanced.

3. On an inhale, lengthen up through the spine as you raise the outside foot to rest on the inner thigh (or calf) of the straight leg. Be sure that neither of you rests the foot on the knee itself; instead, both of you choose a spot above or below the knee.

4. On the exhale, relax the shoulders down and open the knee farther back as you try to create the correct open-hip alignment.

5. Stay here to stabilize further or use an inhale to raise the outside arms overhead and press the palms together overhead.

6. Keep your chest and hips facing forward, your belly firm and your spine lifting.

7. Stay here for at least five breaths before changing to the other leg.

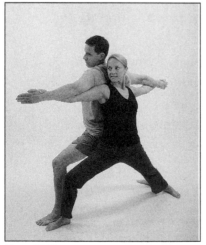

Figure 12.13

Double Warrior

Trust and communication are certainly challenged in this posture, which requires cooperative movement. Balancing and aligning against your partner's back will be frustrating at first, but as you begin to trust and understand one another, movement will flow more smoothly. If you have lots of difficulty keeping your spine, hips and shoulders aligned with your partner, perhaps that is an indication of some postural changes that need to occur in your personal practice (figure 12.13).

1. Stand back to back with your partner, with shoulders and face relaxed. Keep the spine long and the belly firm.

2. Step into a wide stance, with feet about three to four feet apart.

3. Without changing the direction of your hips, look to the front of the room as each partner turns the front foot to face that direction. This will make your feet form a right angle with one another.

4. Raise your arms to shoulder height and link arms with your partner, pressing your palms into your partner's hands to create energy and alignment between your shoulders and back. Keep your balance.

5. Exhale and bend the front knee into Warrior pose, with the thigh trying to get parallel to the ground. Adjust the back foot as you need to, in or out, to achieve the correct posture for the legs. Continue to keep the shoulders, spine, and hips aligned with your partner's.

6. Gaze out over the front hand as you try to stabilize for at least five breaths before switching to the other leg.

Double Crescent

Continue to challenge your strength and flexibility with this partner pose. Remember to always move at your own pace, even if your partner could do more (figure 12.14).

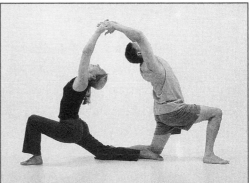

Figure 12.14

1. Face opposite directions in lunge position, using the same leg to lunge for each partner. Make sure your knee is directly over the ankle.

2. Push back through the straight leg to lengthen the leg away from the hip. Then gently lay the knee down to rest on the floor, creating a long backward angle from the hip to the knee. Relax the toes to rest your weight on the top of your foot.

3. Inhale as you balance and raise the arms overhead, lengthening the spine.

4. Exhale as you sink into the hips, still not letting the knee pass the toes.

5. On the next inhale look up toward the extended hands and see if you can create more space upward.

6. On the next exhale, try to relax back so that you've created a long arc in the spine, through the neck, and extending through the arms. If you can, reach back for your partner's hands and let that support guide you farther in the bend.

7. Try to stay here at least three breaths as you attempt to relax back into the pose.

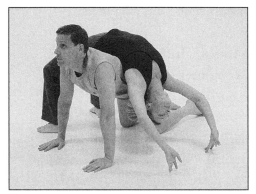

Figure 12.15

Back Massage

The back massage is a safe and supported way to experience the freedom of back bends. The bottom partner experiences benefit as well by strengthening and toning the abs, the arms, and the back. Lots of support and communication are necessary as you develop trust in this posture (figure 12.15).

1. Have one partner rest in all fours (Tabletop), with the hands under the shoulders and the knees under the hips. Engage up and out of the shoulders, firm the belly, and create a flat back, as if you are a sturdy massage table for your partner.

2. The other partner should be standing perpendicular to the "table," with his back to the "table."

3. Sit slowly, adjusting your back, until you are resting on the midback of your partner's flat "table." Keep your feet resting gently on the floor as you extend your arms overhead, and drop the head back to complete the back bend. (If that creates too much strain, then cross your hands over your chest.)

4. The top partner has nothing else to do but breathe and relax as the bottom partner creates the massage effect by rolling the back up on each exhale and rolling the back down on each inhale. The amount of "massage" will be determined by the strength of the "table's" back as he rolls up and down.

5. Try to complete at least five to ten rolls of the back before the top partner comes up very slowly in order to switch positions. If you have trouble getting off the "table," ask the "table" to help by rolling up as you attempt to come off.

Double-Seated Bend

Synchronized breathing is important in this partner posture as you try to use each inhale to lengthen farther outward and each exhale to relax farther downward. If you have very tight hamstrings, feel free to bend the knees slightly to relieve pressure in the legs and back (figure 12.16).

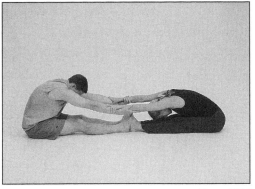

Figure 12.16

1. Sit facing your partner with the bottoms of your feet touching. Keep the legs as straight and strong as you are able.

2. Inhale and lengthen upward through the spine and neck, reaching the arms overhead.

3. On the exhale, begin to hinge at the hips and fold forward toward your partner.

4. Reach for your partner's hands, walking up to wrists or forearms as your legs and back warm and allow you more room to move.

5. Keep your face relaxed and head in the same alignment as the spine as you fold downward. Lead from the chest, and let your arms act as an extension of your long spine.

6. Hold for five or more breaths before releasing hands and rolling up slowly.

Double-Seated Twist

Do this twisting partner pose after you've warmed the back with Double Seated Bend. If you are having trouble reaching your partner's hand, you can always add a strap to assist you (figure 12.17).

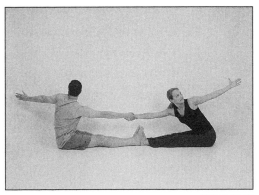

Figure 12.17

1. Sit facing your partner, with the bottoms of your feet touching. Keep the legs as straight and strong as possible.

2. With the back tall, reach across your body to grasp your partner's opposite hand. Relax the shoulder down on the exhale.

3. On the inhale, let the free hand open back, allowing you to twist from the spine and shoulders.

4. Let your gaze follow your hand's movement back, so that the neck is twisting as well. Keep the facial muscles soft and relaxed.

5. Hold here for five breaths, release, and change hands.

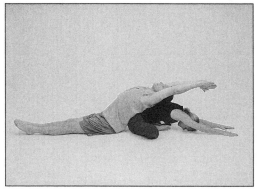

Figure 12.18

Butterfly/Fish

This interdependent partner pose allows one partner to enjoy the hip-opening benefit of Butterfly while the other opens the chest in Fish. The partner in Fish must learn to relax all his weight down onto the Butterfly partner without pushing. The benefit to both partners comes from allowing the weight to rest fully, providing support in opening and assistance in folding. Work on developing an element of trust with this surrender (figure 12.18).

1. Sit with your backs together, spine tall, and shoulders relaxed.

2. Butterfly partner should place the soles of the feet together, and Fish partner should extend the legs straight with feet and knees together.

3. Synchronize the breath so that you are both inhaling to lengthen the spine.

4. On the exhale, Butterfly partner should hinge at the hips and fold forward, walking the hands out as you are able.

5. Fish partner should maintain contact with his partner's back by moving slowly into a back bend. Bring the palms together as you raise the arms overhead to further lengthen the body. Keep the head, shoulders, and back relaxing fully onto your partner. Keep lifting the chest to open the heart.

6. Stay here for at least five breaths before coming back up and changing roles.

Straddle/Fish

Again, this partner pose requires surrender and trust on the part of both partners. The Straddle partner will benefit from the opening of the hips and inside of the legs, while the Fish partner continues to relax, open through the chest, shoulders, and throat (figure 12.19).

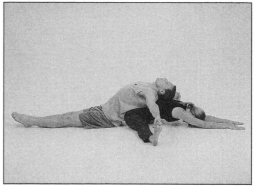

Figure 12.19

1. Sit with your backs firmly touching, spines tall, and shoulders relaxed down.

2. The Straddle partner should slide the legs out to be in a comfortable straddle position, with toes facing up. The Fish partner keeps his legs extended straight, with toes facing up as well.

3. Synchronize the breath and lengthen the spine together on an inhale.

4. On an exhale the Straddle partner hinges from the hips and begins to fold forward, walking the hands outward. Draw the belly toward the floor and then the chest.

5. At the same time, the Fish partner tries to maintain contact with his partner's back as he moves into a gentle back bend.

6. The Fish partner can receive further benefit by opening the arms to the sides and releasing further through the shoulders or perhaps grasping the Straddle partner's feet.

7. Relax fully as you breathe together here for at least five breaths before coming up and reversing roles.

chapter 13

Finding the Reward

Let me be the first to admit that yoga is not the answer to spiritual emptiness. Yoga is not the avenue by which you find peace and fulfillment. Yoga is not even the singular method by which you can enjoy physical and emotional health.

Jesus is.

He is peace. He is joy. He is contentment. He is the only true, lasting path to fulfillment and healing. He is the antidote for spiritual emptiness.

You can find Him in church, in a small group, in Scripture, or any number of places. You can see Him in nature, in childbirth, even in tragedy.

But how about meeting God, really spending quality time with Him . . . on your *mat*? . . . Letting your mat become a sacred place where you listen to His whisper? . . . Using time on your mat to focus your thoughts into coherent, meaningful prayer? . . . Letting your practice be another opportunity to worship, this time without distraction or interruption? . . . Creating emotional health that releases you from stress and anxiety? . . . Restoring your body to the healthy, vibrant system God created, free of pain, able to move and serve?

Your mat can't do it alone. It is not a magic carpet on which you are miraculously transformed. But it is a vehicle, when coupled with a Christ-centered intention, that can draw you to the foot of the Cross.

Your quiet, reflective, healing yoga practice can bring you into the relationship that does offer ultimate peace, unconditional love, unending joy, and eternal rewards.

Be ready for a change—a life-changing transformation!

Inhale the power of God in which you can do all things through Christ.

Exhale the words, attitudes, and values that can change the world.

Notes

Chapter 1—Why "Christian Yoga"?

1. Matt Redman, *Facedown* (Lottbridge Drove, Eastbourne, England: Kingsway Communications, 2004), 17.

2. www.christianitytoday.com, Agnieszka Tennant, "Yes to Yoga," / (19 May 2005).

3. Joyce Rupp, *The Cup of Our Life* (Notre Dame, Ind.: Ave Maria Press, 1997), 50.

Chapter 2—Getting Started

1. Tilden Edwards, *Living in the Presence* (San Francisco: Harper, 1987), 18.

Chapter 3—Connecting the Breath

1. Richard Foster, *Meditative Prayer* (Madison, Wis.: InterVarsity, 1983), 21.

2. Tom Ryan, *Prayer of Heart and Body* (Mahwah, N.J.: Paulist Press, 1995), 66.

3. The breathing techniques described in this section are adapted from Richard Rosen, "Inhale, Exhale, Relax," *Yoga Journal Balanced Living* (Winter 2004), 93–98.

Chapter 4—Getting Warm

1. Wayne Cordeiro, *Rising Above* (Ventura, Calif.: Regal, 2004), 72.

2. Nancy Roth, *An Invitation to Christian Yoga* (Boston: Cowley, 1989, 2001), 23.

Chapter 5—Finding Focus (Balance Postures)

1. Joanna Weaver, *Having a Mary Heart in a Martha World* (Colorado Springs: Waterbrook, 2000), 99–100.

2. Bill Hybels, *Too Busy Not to Pray* (Downer's Grove, Ill.: InterVarsity, 1988, 1998), 125.

Chapter 6—Drawing Strength (Standing Postures)

1. Rick Warren, *The Purpose Driven Life: What on Earth Am I Here For?* (Grand Rapids: Zondervan, 2002), 272.

Chapter 8—Achieving Rest

1. Max Lucado, *Traveling Light* (Nashville: W Publishing Group, 2001), 4–5.

2. Robert Benson, *Living Prayer* (New York: Putnam, 1998), 27.

Chapter 9—Hearing the Whisper

1. Claire Cloninger, *The Kaleidoscope* (Waco: Word, 1988), 102.

2. Matt Redman, *Facedown* (Lottbridge Drove, Eastbourne, England: Kingsway Communications, 2004), 97.

3. Richard Foster, *Meditative Prayer* (Madison, Wis.: InterVarsity, 1983), 8–10.

4. John Ortberg, *The Life You've Always Wanted* (Grand Rapids: Zondervan, 1997, 2002), 178.

5. Ibid.

6. Robert Benson, *Living Prayer*, 110.

Chapter 10—Creating a Flow (Linking the Postures)

1. Baron Baptiste, *Journey into Power*, 53.

Chapter 11—Involving Your Children

1. Facts from the American Obesity Association at www.obesity.org and from Childhood Mental Health at www.childhooddisorders.com.

Chapter 12—Connecting with a Partner

1. Cain Carroll and Lori Kimata, *Partner Yoga* (New York: Rodale, 2000), 35.

VISIT

www.christianyoga.us